Author Note

The subject of this book is variously referred to as Sundowning, Sundowners, Sundown Syndrome, Sundowning Syndrome, Sundowner Syndrome, Sundowner's Syndrome, and Hospital Psychosis. For consistency, throughout this book, we use the names *Sundowner's Syndrome* and *Sundowners*, except in quotes from medical research articles in which we use the terminology ascribed by the article's author.

* * * * * * *

The caregiver quotes used throughout this book have been drawn from the many hundreds of caregiver comments posted at the Sundownerfacts.com website, which have been anonymized to protect the identity of the posting caregiver. Hopefully, they give some insight into Sundowner's Syndrome—what it is, its symptoms, and the fears and frustrations of those who care for a patient with Sundowners. And people continue to come to the website daily to leave comments, ask specific questions, vent, or offer advice they have found helpful in their own journey with the disease. Thank you all for your willingness to share your wisdom, insights and frustrations with others who are seeking understanding and help in dealing with Sundowners patients. It is because so many people frequent the website searching for help and information on Sundowners that this Sundowner's Syndrome Caregiver Guide has been written.

SUNDOWNER'S SYNDROME

A Caregiver Guide

from
Sundownerfacts.com

Introduction by
Liz Barlowe, CMC.

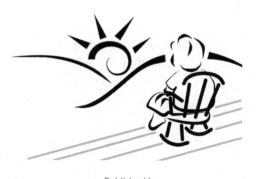

Published by
iSight Technologies

iSight Technologies
P.O Box 547896
Orlando, Florida, 32854

ISBN: 978-0-9859474-0-8

Library of Congress Control Number: 2012948565

Design and Typesetting by
Geoff Benge at
Silver Fern Bookworks

Printed in the United States

Contents

Introduction 7

1. *What is Sundowner's Syndrome?* 9

2. *Medication* 19

3. *Some Approaches to Try* 43

4. *Family Dynamics* 55

5. *Caregiver Well-Being* 71

6. *Resources* 83

7. *Pay It Forward* 93

Appendix. *Drug Chart* 101

Introduction

Liz Barlowe, CMC.

SUNDOWNER'S SYNDROME A CAREGIVER GUIDE successfully explores the challenges that Sundowner's Syndrome presents to caregivers and shares effective strategies to help minimize or alleviate symptoms. The guide comprises a comprehensive compilation of approaches on how to effectively care for individuals experiencing Sundowner's Syndrome. It is a practical book that illustrates the importance of sharing information with others in an effort to relieve the suffering of those with Sundowners. Much of the material in this guide is drawn from the experience of people on the frontlines—caregivers dealing with the daily challenges Sundowner's Syndrome presents. Their entries are creative and compassionate, giving hope to readers who might be thinking the situation hopeless.

As a professional geriatric care manager, I have consulted with many clients over the years who have struggled with caring for a loved one demonstrating Sundowners symptoms. As if the diagnosis of dementia isn't enough, it is often compounded by extreme changes in personality around late afternoon to early evening. What has consistently struck me is the caregiver's strength and perseverance given this difficult situation. Day after day most caregivers continue to try new approaches to combat the challenging behavior brought on by Sundowners. I have learned as much from these caregivers and their willingness to try different strategies as they have from my guidance.

Caregivers are the innovators of effective treatments for Sundowner's Syndrome, and I am confident that by implementing some or all of the strategies outlined in this guide they will compassionately help the loved ones under their care. This book is filled with a wide variety of strategies proven to help minimize the effects of Sundowner's Syndrome. As readers experiment they will find some of the strategies work brilliantly while others may have little effect on their patient.

Finally, the need to share caregiver expertise is imperative for the benefit of all who deal with this health crisis. I urge caregivers to post their experiences on *Sundownerfacts.com* or other such websites so that we can all share what works and what does not in mitigating the symptoms of Sundowner's Syndrome.

1

What is Sundowner's Syndrome?

PEOPLE WHO CARE FOR patients with Sundowner's Syndrome often liken their experience to entering the 'twilight zone.' At first glance, Sundowners sounds like fiction—people becoming irrational, violent and abusive around sunset, and then, the following morning, being unable to remember anything odd about their behavior. Many caregivers are confused when they first encounter Sundowner's Syndrome, a fact borne out by comments such as this one.

"My grandmother has Parkinson's disease. Recently, she has been getting paranoid at night. She constantly thinks people are looking in her windows at night, shining flashlights at her, trying to break in. She panics and turns her alarm on a lot. The neighbors never see anything; nothing has ever been found to show there is any fact to what she believes she is seeing at night. Is it possible that this is a problem stemming from her Parkinson's disease, or is it something else?"

Once the reality of these symptoms set in, caregivers normally swing into action and seek information. They soon discover there is very little guidance available for this condition. In fact, of the over twenty-one million citations of biomedical research articles in the *National Center for Biotechnology Information* database (see Chapter 6 for more information on this database), less than twenty-five refer to Sundowner's Syndrome. One of the most recent research articles on Sundowners in this database is titled *Sundown Syndrome in Persons With Dementia: An Update*. This lengthy research article, written by N. Khachiyants, D. Trinkle, S.J. Son, and K.Y. Kim, is actually a meta-study of all previous studies undertaken on the subject and provides perhaps the best overview of Sundowner's Syndrome currently available. And since it is such a trove of helpful information, we will refer to this study numerous times throughout this book.

Sundowner's Syndrome—A Definition

According to the *Sundown Syndrome in Persons With Dementia: An Update* study, *"Sundowning in demented individuals, as distinct clinical phenomena, is still open to debate in terms of clear definition, etiology, operationalized parameters, validity of clinical construct, and interventions. In general, sundown syndrome is characterized by the emergence or increment of neuropsychiatric symptoms such as agitation, confusion, anxiety, and aggressiveness in late afternoon, in the evening, or at night."*

In short, Sundowner's Syndrome is the name given to an ailment that causes symptoms of confusion around or after 'sundown.' These symptoms appear in people who suffer from Alzheimer's disease or other forms of dementia. However, not all patients who suffer from dementia or Alzheimer's exhibit the symptoms of Sundowner's Syndrome. Conversely, some people exhibit symptoms of

dementia throughout the day which grow worse in the late afternoon and evening, while others may exhibit virtually no symptoms at all until the sun goes down.

Sundowner's Syndrome largely remains a mystery to medical science, although there are several theories about why these
symptoms begin at night. Several studies are currently being conducted to try to determine the exact cause of Sundowners. In
the meantime, there is a broad range of divergent opinion within
the medical community as to its cause. Some doctors believe it
results from an accumulation of sensory stimulation throughout
the day that begins to overwhelm and stress a patient. Other doctors speculate that Sundowner's Syndrome is caused by hormonal
imbalances that occur at night. And still others believe that the
onset of the symptoms at night is due to simple fatigue, or to factors such as medications given in the morning wearing off as the
day goes on. Social patterns may also contribute, since sundown
is typically associated with lifelong patterns of transition such as
returning from work, awaiting the arrival of a spouse from work,
cooking dinner, and the like. A person may grow restless or agitated because of this sense of transition, feeling they need to go
home, or awaiting the arrival of someone. There are also those
who believe that Sundowner's Syndrome has to do with the anxiety
caused by light patterns and an inability to see as well in the dark.

The theory that the symptoms have something to do with dark-
ness has been supported by studies that show the symptoms sub-
side within an hour of the return of daylight. There is also some
evidence that nursing facility patients show an increase in Sundowners' symptoms during winter, which may suggest some affin-
ity with Seasonal Affective Disorder (SAD), a disorder believed
to cause depression in the winter due to the shorter periods of
sunlight which affects people of all ages.

Currently, there is no definitive test for Sundowner's Syndrome. A diagnosis is made through observation of the patient. In the majority of instances, the patient is unaware of his or her behavior and the effect it is having on those around them. The distinguishing feature of Sundowner's Syndrome symptoms is their timing component; Sundowners occurs around the time the sun goes down—late afternoon—and on into the night. During the day, the symptoms are not typically present. It is this timing issue that often alerts caregivers to the diagnosis.

The following posts demonstrate how this timing issue plays out.

"My mom is 75 years old and I can't be sure what is wrong with her as after 6:00 in the evening I can see a change when I try to explain things to her. She can't understand anything I try to tell her. She starts telling me things that happened back when she was a child, and doesn't remember what she was talking about. Sometimes I get so frustrated I have to leave the room to gather my wits and she starts crying or just pouts. She has chores to do and one chore in particular is doing the dishes. Each night when she unloads the dishwasher, she either puts the dishes in places where they don't belong or forgets where she puts them. She seems okay when she sees her doctor and says she is just fine. She hates it when I tell him what she is doing."

"I have an 86 year old mother whom I live with and take care of. For the past few months, her hallucinations have been getting worse at night, and I am woken up every night with her calling for me in fear. She sees people in her room. Children on her bed playing, and last night, she was sitting

on the edge of her bed saying she was lost. She is from England, and she thought she was over there, and lost. I have to convince her in a very calm way that she is safe and okay."

"My mom is very alert in the day, but as night comes, she starts with the frustration, crying, anger, talking to herself for very long periods of time, and then in the middle of the night...seeing things. I am so tired; I don't know what to do."

"My mother just turned 84. In the past several weeks, she has started with the sundowning behavior. I'm really sorry for any of you whose loved one has this syndrome. It's just awful, and you know by watching the person that they have to be miserable. The constant babbling, the constant movement, irritation, confusion, hallucinations—I never get to sleep. It starts about 5:30–6:00 P.M. and goes until almost 7:00 A.M., sometimes later. It's the most amazing thing I've ever seen— she is a completely different person at night. Frail during the day, and King Kong at night! It's trying, it's tiring, and it's extremely difficult to watch your loved one go through it. And it requires more patience than I ever knew I had."

"My grandfather is almost 83. He suffers from Sundowner's Syndrome. He has had Alzheimer's for almost three years now and, just recently, it has gotten worse. He is very forgetful of everything during the day. When the sun goes down and it gets dark, that's when my grandpa wants to go 'home,' but he is at home. This is when he forgets who my grandmother is and he gets very abusive. We took his car and license away almost two years ago but he still tries to get in the car, and if he does get in the car, he will sit there *for hours at a time. If you try to tell him to come back inside, he will yell at you or curse at you. My grandfather is a very religious man and never in his 83 years has he talked the way he does now. Why is that? Why does he want to go 'home' when it gets dark?"*

"Forget about sleeping all night. If I can even get three hours of uninterrupted sleep in a night, I feel like I have won the jackpot. Our biggest problem is kind of funny when reviewed in the daylight. My husband hears music and wants the radio turned off. When I tell him there is no radio on, he gets mad and calls me a liar. From there, he gets more and more upset and angry because I am so selfish as to keep him awake all night by listening to loud music. He lies in bed and screams, 'Unplug it. Unplug It,' every few minutes. Then he starts making childish threats like wetting his pants. The whole thing must be very frustrating for him."

Many caregivers also report that their Sundowner's Syndrome patients exhibit extra bursts of energy and astonishing strength at night.

"One of my sisters told me about Sundowner's Syndrome. I believe with all my heart that my mother has this. She can wake at 5:00 A.M. and go all day. And when the sun goes down, she has more energy than sixteen mules. She is up all night. That is when she is most likely to wander off somewhere. She reminds me of the rabbit on the commercial—she just keeps going and going."

"I think my mom is in the beginning stages of Sundowners. She had a stroke nine years ago which killed her kidneys

and she has been on dialysis for eight years. She just started doing some weird things in the last two weeks. The waking up at night is definitely one of them. She wants to take a shower and get ready, even though it's one-thirty in the morning. She also seems to do physical things that normally she cannot do. She opened a heavy sliding glass door and walked out to the backyard and fell down. We were looking for her all over the house and couldn't find her. Finally we went out to the backyard and saw her sitting on the grass asking for someone to help her. I just couldn't believe it! All I kept saying was how did she get out there?"

Sundowner's Syndrome symptoms can also develop suddenly, which often takes caregivers off guard.

"Tragically, from my experience, the onset is quick and this is one of the reasons that makes this condition so hard to deal with. The rapid decline intermixed with times of clarity is so hard to fathom. The only bit of good news in my mother's case is that it can diminish and there are times when things are relatively okay. But I have found that this is not an indication of a reversal; it's more of an ebb and flow type situation."

"I have a very close friend who was just diagnosed with Sundowner's Syndrome. He is 88 and lost his wife about two years ago. He has had some health issues, but with the right medicines, he was clear thinking and aptly used the computer. My question is how long is the onset? Is it possible to have no symptoms and, within a few weeks, be full-blown Sundowners? He was fine when I spent a week with him

*about a month ago and we communicated daily by email.
Now he is evidently incoherent a lot of the time. Somehow
this just doesn't sound right..."*

*"We are just experiencing what the staff told us is 'Sundown-
ing'. My mom is 95 and two weeks ago, she was going out
to lunch once a week and living alone and doing all her
own cooking, etc. Her delight was trips to shop or just 'poke'
around as she said. With the hot weather, she was not feeling
like eating and was not drinking water either. Her sodium
level fell dangerously low and she had to be hospitalized
and given an IV. Three days later, her levels were all normal
and she went to rehab because she was so physically weak.
She is fine during the day, but by 5:00 P.M. at night, she is
violent and screaming and does not want anyone near her.
It is so unlike her as she has always been gentle and sweet."*

*"My father who is 73 years old has been suffering from Par-
kinson's disease for seven years now, and Sundowner's Syndrome for a few months. It kicked in full force with no warnings. No sleep for anyone at night. My sister, wife and I have
been taking turns watching him at night so my mother, who
cares for him during the day, can sleep. He wanders, forgets
to use his walker or forgets how to use it. He tells me to take
him home, even though he is home. He calls me his brother
John, who has been dead since 1972. Apparently, there is
nothing out there to treat this problem, or so I have been
told. Sleeping medicine works against him and causes him
to become more confused. We are wearing thin on all fronts
and it appears that the final option is a nursing home or
paying for private care."*

There also appears to be a strong correlation between hospitalization, surgeries, urinary tract infections and the onset of Sundowner's Syndrome. Hospital delirium is a well-documented complication of hospitalization for many older adults, characterized by sudden confusion and inattention. This may be the first time a person exhibits signs of Sundowner's Syndrome or a person with some symptoms may experience the exacerbation of symptoms. Although delirium has generally been thought to be transient and reversible, many patients seem to suffer an ongoing decline. Infections, medications, and physical trauma are often associated with delirium in older adults. Many caregivers have posted comments on the website pointing out this connection, and we will revisit this topic in the following chapter on medication. For now, this post from a caregiver illustrates the point.

"My grandfather was just diagnosed with congestive heart failure. He has been in the hospital for about five days. Last night he started acting really paranoid. He didn't believe he was in a real hospital; he thought the whole thing was a scam. Today he was talking about being kidnapped. When I alerted the nurse, she tried to tell me that people of his age get confused and that it's normal. I'm thinking that this nurse is an idiot. He was just fine the day before yesterday; he understood where he was and why he was there. Now it's like him against the world. I just don't understand what has happened! Can dementia just creep up on you like that? This is so hard to understand. He is one of the most level-headed men I know and now he is being totally irrational. He did a 180 in a matter of two days."

As we have already mentioned in this chapter, Sundowner's Syndrome is not a focal point for ongoing medical research. What information is available is spotty at best, and often hard to find. Yet it is of vital importance for anyone who has a family member with Sundowner's Syndrome or is a caregiver for such a person to have the most accurate and up-to-date information available. As a result, this book attempts to present the substantiated facts along with the caregiving best practices that are currently available. However, we also realize that some of the best advice for dealing with patients with Sundowner's Syndrome comes from those who are currently, or have in the past been in the 'trenches' providing such care. So throughout this book we have interwoven the facts and information together with the best anecdotal caregiving tips and insights posted on the website. Our hope is that by doing so, you will find this book informative and supportive in your journey caring for a patient suffering from Sundowner's Syndrome.

2

Medication

"DOES ANYONE WHO HAS a mother with Sundowner's Syndrome have any advice about medication and something that has been effective for a loved one? I would appreciate any advice. We are at the beginning stages of all this..."

"Mom had partial knee surgery three months ago and has never been the same. She has to be restrained, falls, and now the doctor says it's Sundowner's Syndrome. Around 3–4 P.M. everyday, she starts taking the blankets off her bed, her socks, sees things, and the like. Will she ever come home to her house again? She knows all of us, talks about her parents (deceased) and wants to go see them. I am at a loss...what medications do we need for her?"

The most often repeated concern among the many posts from caregivers relates to medication: What is available? What works? What doesn't work? And what does over-medication or under-medication look like? The variety of responses to these concerns illustrates the extreme difficulty the caregivers of patients with Sundowner's Syndrome face in managing the condition and finding solutions.

Perhaps we should not be surprised that medication is one of the biggest concerns for these caregivers. We live in a modern world where there seems to be a drug or pill for every malady; surely there must be an effective drug for treating Sundowner's Syndrome. Unfortunately, it's not that simple.

But before we dig deeper into the area of medication, it should be pointed out that this caregiver guide is not meant to be an expert treatise on the subject. *The information provided here is solely for the purpose of education and should not be construed as medical advice.* What follows is a compilation of the available information on medications and treatments related to Sundowner's Syndrome. Its purpose is to provide caregivers with an overview and starting point for discussions with health care providers. As a caregiver, you should seek advice from your medical practitioner or locate a professional experienced in medications for dementia and Sundowners. You are your patient's advocate and you should prepare a list of concerns and questions, along with carefully monitoring their progress and/or any side effects they may experience from the medications they are taking.

That said, there are no drugs currently being used exclusively for the treatment of Sundowner's Syndrome. Instead, patients who have Sundowners are normally treated with an array of medications that are used more generally with dementia. The *Sundown Syndrome in Persons With Dementia: An Update* report, to which we referred in the previous chapter, states, "hypnotics, benzodiazepines, and low-potency antipsychotics are among the conventional therapy that is used to manage evening agitation and behavioral disruptions associated with sundowning."

The following is an overview of these categories of medications along with some of the common concerns and important information for caregivers to consider.

Hypnotics

The primary function of this class of drugs (also called soporifics) is to induce sleep. They are used in the treatment of insomnia, and in surgical anesthesia. The names of drugs in this class include eszopiclone (Lunesta), zaleplon (Zonata), zolpidem (Ambien, Ambien CR), and zopiclone (Imovane in Canada, Australia and Zimovane in the UK). Medical research suggests that these drugs should only be prescribed for a few days at the lowest effective dose, and whenever possible, avoided altogether in the elderly. For further details, you can refer to the research paper, *Drug the Bull*, which can be viewed at the following website, *www.ncbi.nlm.nih. gov/pubmed/15587763.*

Benzodiazepines

Xanax, Paxal, Rivotril, Valium, Restoril, and Halcion are all benzodiazepines targeted to enhance the effect of neurotransmitters in the brain, which results in sedative, hypnotic (sleep-inducing), anxiolytic (anti-anxiety), anticonvulsant, muscle relaxant and amnesic action. These properties make benzodiazepines useful in treating anxiety, insomnia, agitation, seizures, muscle spasms, and alcohol withdrawal.

Antipsychotics

The list of drugs in this class is rather long: haloperidol (Haldol, Serenace), droperidol (Droleptan), chlorpromazine (Thorazine, Largactil), fluphenazine (Prolixin), perphenazine (Trilafon), prochlorperazine (Compazine), thioridazine (Mellaril, Melleril), trifluoperazine (Stelazine), mesoridazine (Serentil), pericyazine (Amplan), promazine (Sparine), triflupromazine (Vesprin), levomepromazine (Nozinan), Promethazine (Phenergan), pimozide (Orap), cyamemazine (Tercian), chlorprothixene (Cloxan, Taractan, Truxal), clopenthixol (Sordinol), flupenthixol (Depixol, Fluanxol), thiothixene (Navane), zuclopenthixol (Cisordinol, Zyprexa, Risperdal), quetiapine (Seroquel), ziprasidone (Geodon), amisulpride (Solian, Sulpitac, Amitrex, Soltus, Amazeo), asenapine (Saphris), paliperidone (Invega), iloperidone (Fanapt, Fanapta, and previously known as Zomaril), zotepine (Nipolept, Losizopilon, Lodopin, Setous), sertindole (Serdolect, Serlect), and lurasidone (Latuda).

Antipsychotic drugs are tranquilizing psychiatric medications that are mainly used to manage psychosis, delusions, hallucinations, schizophrenia and bipolar disorder. Many antipsychotics carry a 'black box' warning, meaning that the description of the drug appears inside a black box on the label, and also on any advertising for the drug. This is the strongest warning the FDA uses to alert doctors and patients to the dangers of a particular drug. These 'black box' drugs can be particularly dangerous to elderly patients. For further reading on this issue, check out the article at the following website: *www.bipolar.about.com/od/ antipsychotics/a/1blackbox.htm.*

In addition, antipsychotics are increasingly used to treat nonpsychotic disorders. In the United States, new drugs are tested in clinical trials before they are approved for use in the general public. These clinical trials are carried out to prove that the drug is effective in treating a certain medical condition and demonstrate that the drug works in the way it was designed to and is safe when used as directed. The drug label gives information about the drug, including the approved dosage and how it is to be given to treat the medical condition for which it has been approved. When a drug is used in a way that is different from that described in the FDA-approved drug label, it is called 'off-label' use. This can mean that the drug is used for a different disease or medical condition, or given in a different dosage than is recommended. Off-label use is also called 'non-approved' or 'unapproved' use of a drug. Almost all antipsychotic drugs used to treat patients with Sundowner's Syndrome are prescribed off-label.

The side effects of antipsychotic drugs are serious and include many things that could also contribute to the advancement of symptoms in patients with dementia. Elderly people with dementia are at risk from serious and life-threatening side effects when treated with antipsychotics. Research indicates there is an increased risk of stroke, and a small increased risk of death when antipsychotics are used in the treatment of elderly people with dementia.

In 2011, the *New York Times* wrote a scathing exposé on the use of off-label antipsychotic drugs on dementia patients. The article begins:

"Nearly one in seven elderly nursing home residents, nearly all of them with dementia, are given powerful atypical antipsychotic drugs even though the medicines increase the risks of death and are not approved for such treatments, a government audit found...

Government, taxpayers, nursing home residents as well as their families and caregivers should be outraged and seek solutions," Daniel R. Levinson, inspector general of the Department of Health and Human Services, wrote in announcing the audit results.

Mr. Levinson noted that such drugs—which include Risperdal, Zyprexa, Seroquel, Abilify and Geodon—are 'potentially lethal' to many of the patients getting them and that some drug manufacturers illegally marketed their medicines for these uses "putting profits before safety."

You can read the full text of the article on the *New York Times* website at the following web address: *www.nytimes.com/2011/05/10/health/policy/10drug.html*.

Another recent article in the *British Medical Journal* assessed the mortality risks associated with individual antipsychotic drugs including aripiprazole, haloperidol, olanzapine, quetiapine, risperidone and ziprasidone. You can read the full text of the article at the following website: *www.bmj.com/press-releases/2012/02/22/specific-antipsychotic-drugs-increase-risk-death-elderly-dementia-patients*.

With this in mind, let's take a look at some of the problems and the advice caregivers have offered to resolve those problems. These have been grouped in the form of observations. The observations are not meant to be a substitute for sound medical advice, but are merely an anecdotal compilation of what other caregivers have seen and experienced in relation to medicating patients with Sundowner's Syndrome.

Observation One: There is no one drug or combination of drugs that will always help a patient with Sundowner's Syndrome. One person's answer to a prayer is another's nightmare.

The website comments related to medication are filled with desperate pleas for help and seemingly contradictory information on the use of drugs for treating Sundowners patients. To illustrate, we have assembled a number of comments below on just one drug, haloperidol, which is sold under the trade name Haldol. However, Haldol carries a black box label; it is prescribed off-label to control the symptoms of Sundowner's Syndrome in the elderly. In fact, the FDA's website *(www.fda.gov/Drugs)* carries this warning regarding haloperidol: "Studies have shown that older adults with dementia (a brain disorder that affects the ability to remember, think clearly, communicate, and perform daily activities and that may cause changes in mood and personality) who take antipsychotics (medications for mental illness) such as haloperidol have an increased chance of death during treatment . . .The Food and Drug Administration (FDA) does not approve haloperidol for the treatment of behavior problems in older adults with dementia. Talk to the doctor who prescribed this medication if you, a family member, or someone you care for has dementia and is taking haloperidol."

The FDA website goes on to inform us that haloperidol "is used to treat psychotic disorders (conditions that cause difficulty telling the difference between things or ideas that are real and things or ideas that are not real). Haloperidol is also used to control motor tics (uncontrollable need to repeat certain body movements) and verbal tics (uncontrollable need to repeat sounds or words) in adults and children who have Tourette's disorder (a condition characterized by motor or verbal tics) . . . Haloperidol is in a group of medications called conventional antipsychotics. It works by decreasing abnormal excitement in the brain."

With this as background, let's look at a sampling of posted comments regarding Haldol. First, we will review some negative comments, followed by some positive ones.

"My late husband had dementia and Sundowners. The doctor put him on Haldol and it made him worse. Aricept is [a] much better [medication for him] and he didn't have the falling down that went with Haldol."

"Please, no one should use Haldol [a] terrible medicine [with] terrible side effects. My mother, at 88, had [Haldol] for two days in hospital and she went crazy for weeks, not just saying crazy [things], went crazy. We finally could not handle her, put her in a nursing home and finally, after six weeks, she just woke up and said, 'Why am I here and what happened to me?' Like a light bulb—on and off. She did not even know her name, went into paranoid states and had to be restrained at times. She would scream for everyone to help her; that we and the nurses were trying to kill her. She slept all day, came alive at night, had to be force fed and diapered. [She] would not keep her clothes on and rocked on her bed on her hands and knees. Never in my life have I seen a medicine affect someone like that. Research this medicine; it is not for normal elderly people.... I found out later [Haldol] has terrible side effects in the elderly and is really used to subdue people in mental wards."

"I am a nurse [who] cared for a man on Haldol. The Haldol was the cause of his hallucinations. Once he was off that medication, he was alert."

"I just had a call from my mom's hospice case nurse. Mom is 95 and the nurse told me that although a doctor had signed the script for Haldol, in her experience (over 40 years of hospice nursing), this drug was dangerous in the elderly."

In contrast:

"My grandfather was on Ativan and Risperadol, and they had a horrible adverse effect on him. The only medication that gave him some help, not a lot but some, was Haldol."

"Haldol seems to be working for her so far. She is sleeping longer hours with short 'potty breaks' that are not disturbing to anyone but her, and...she does not remember them the next day."

"We are using Haldol for my mom, as well as a Xanax earlier in the day, and in the morning when she wakes up. Her Sundowners [symptoms] last from about 6:00 P.M. to 8:00 A.M. She also takes Trazadone. Her confusion is not gone, or really a lot better; she just sleeps more steadily and is not up and worried as much during the night. Mom has progressed quickly the last few months and it is taking me and my siblings by surprise at how fast things are moving. One thing I will add, my mom did not do well on the Exelon patch. It works different for everyone."

"I want to thank the lady who worked with dementia patients in the hospital. She suggested Haldol, and when hospice came in, we got Haldol for my mother-in-law. All the depression medication did not help, the anxiety pills did not help, but Haldol did. I actually got to have a small conversation with her. It didn't last too long, but the yelling and screaming and night terrors have slowed way down. My mother-in-law has since passed, but we cannot say enough about Haldol.... What a difference the right medicine made."

"The right medicines work wonders.... Granny was scream-
ing all night and day and had night terrors all day. I was
crying, she was crying. [When] hospice came in and saw
what was happening, [they suggested] Haldol. Given cor-
rectly for three days, I started to see a difference...it was
easier. [Finally]...she was almost sane again.... Get the right
medication. Good luck."

And a final comment that says it all.

"Interesting how each medication works differently on dif-
ferent people. I just wish there was a cure...sighs with wish-
ful thinking..."

Just reading these comments is enough to give a person
whiplash! Can everyone be talking about the same drug? Yes,
they are. This illustrates why Sundowner's Syndrome is so
incredibly difficult to get a handle on. Drugs that work for one
patient do not appear to work for another. From these caregiver
observations, it would seem that the best course of action is
to proceed with caution, making sure that any changes in prescription medications are carefully monitored by a medical
professional experienced in this area and who is ready to make
adjustments when necessary. Seek out medical professionals
who are experienced in geriatrics and dementia, and who will
take the time to explain to you the potential risks and benefits
of a particular medicine.

Observation Two: Even drugs that appear to work well at alleviating the symptoms of Sundowner's Syndrome can stop working within a short period of time.

Perhaps the worst feeling is thinking that you have finally found an effective medication for your patient's Sundowners symptoms, and then realizing that after a period of time—a remarkably short period for some patients—that medication is no longer effective. That has been the experience of the following caregivers.

"Here is an update about my November 5 Ambien CR recommendation: After only three weeks of using [the medication], its effectiveness has diminished from eight hour to four or five hours, sometimes less. My mother-in-law (95) now goes to bed at 9:00 P.M. after taking the Ambien CR at 8:45. She is usually up again at 2:00 A.M. And it is taking longer and longer to take effect. Initially, within fifteen minutes, she was relaxing and getting drowsy. Now she can be still wide-awake after an hour of taking the Ambien. So I am back at square one and am getting up three or four times a night with her."

"My husband and I moved out of our house and into my parents' home to care for my dad. He is getting increasingly worse which keeps him up all night talking, yelling at people, trying to get out of bed.... I find myself up every twenty minutes making sure he's okay.... Our doctor prescribed a sleep medication, which worked for about two weeks and now...it's not working at all!"

"Check with your provider regarding the long time use of medication like Ativan. They can lose their effectiveness after only two weeks."

Observation Three: It is very difficult to determine if a medication is making a patient's symptoms better or worse.

To complicate matters, patients with Sundowner's Syndrome normally have a variety of other medical conditions that require medication. For example, many Sundowners patients also have Alzheimer's or Parkinson's disease, high blood pressure or even diabetes for which they are treated with drugs. And since Sundowners rarely occurs alone, it becomes extremely difficult to decide which treatments are effective.

And then there is the question of the side effects of potent drugs on frail, elderly patients. This is an issue that concerns many caregivers. So let's continue looking at the drug Haldol, (though any number of other antipsychotics would illustrate the point just as effectively). The following is a list of the potential side effects of Haldol as noted on the FDA website.

"Haloperidol may cause side effects. Tell your doctor if any of these symptoms are severe or do not go away: Drowsiness; dry mouth; increased saliva; blurred vision; loss of appetite; constipation; diarrhea; heartburn; nausea; vomiting; difficulty falling asleep or staying asleep; blank facial expression; uncontrollable eye movements; unusual, slowed, or uncontrollable movements of any part of the body; restlessness; agitation; nervousness; mood changes; dizziness; headache; breast enlargement or pain; decreased sexual ability in men; increased sexual desire; difficulty urinating."

All of these side effects are serious, and it is very difficult to get an elderly patient with Sundowner's Syndrome to articulate such changes in their bodies. Are they, for example, able to tell the caregiver that they feel dizzy, or nauseous? And many of these potential side effects are actually the same as the symptoms of the condition the drug is attempting to ameliorate; restlessness, agitation, mood changes, difficulty falling asleep or staying asleep. These are all stressful symptoms of Sundowner's Syndrome. Perhaps this helps to illuminate why some Sundowners patients who took Haldol improved while others became worse. Those who got worse may have been experiencing some of the known side effects of the drug.

Observation Four: A patient's condition needs to be treated holistically with an awareness of overmedicating and the balance of benefits to risk.

By now you may be feeling a sense of despair; that's understandable. There is no conclusive evidence as to the overall effect drug therapies have on patients with Sundowner's Syndrome. As well, some caregivers have serious concerns about their patients being overmedicated. They report frustration at the sheer number of drugs being prescribed and the dire effect this can have on their Sundowners patient. Note the frustration and anger evident in these posts on the issue.

"While [mom] was in the rehab center, the doctor prescribed a total of twelve prescriptions, in addition to the five she was already taking. I refuse to continue all twelve medications. I have made an appointment with her primary care physician to gradually wean her off [these drugs]. Because of all the medications, she's stuttering, is angrier and more agitated, and acting stubbornly. All she wants to do is sleep."

"Over the last three years, dad has become more like an Alzheimer's victim. Memory loss, some stroke-like speech

loss, dressing muck ups, and finally we are seeing Sundowner's Syndrome. And he was on medication for heart problems...Atenolol, and Metformin for diabetes, plus various other medications. Yes, I think the entire world is overmedicated. Doctors seem to prescribe drugs and make referrals to other doctors. I think they are becoming less and less able to actually heal anyone. It is sickening and frustrating. And once you are put on a medication, it is very difficult to remove you from it. No doctor wants to remove anyone from a medication they are currently taking."

"Make sure your patient is not over-medicated, which happened in my mom's case. She went from the ability to feed herself to not being able to after a hospitalization where she was loaded up with unneeded drugs. After another hospitalization, when she was weaned off those drugs, she was again able to feed herself."

"My father has dementia and was getting very violent at night and walking around all night long. A psychiatric nurse suggested that it could be the Ambien the doctor had prescribed for him. So we took him off it, and in three days he was a normal, sweet man again. Now I don't know if it was the combination of drugs with the Ambien, as he was also on Risperidone, Hydralazine, Metoprolol, and Mirtazapine (Remeron). We are in the process of trying to wean him off some of these with the help of the psychiatric nurse. All these doctors just dope these people up. It's terrible."

"My mother was diagnosed with vascular dementia four years ago. I have been the only caregiver for years. She is 86 and has been in the hospital for four weeks awaiting placement in a nursing home. Her Sundowners symptoms have started again. Unknown to me, the hospital put her on Haldol (three doses). Her daytime agitation got worse and three days later, it was as if she had Parkinson's. The doctor refuses to admit [that this] was [caused by] the drug. Her symptoms of Parkinson's have subsided (ten days later). Last night her Sundowners acted up, and guess what? The doctor prescribed Ambien and Haldol! I went to the hospital at 1:30 A.M. and stayed until 3:00 A.M. and I gave her Melatonin, which had helped at home. How can I get the hospital to stop giving her drugs with definite black box warnings? The medical profession needs to realize that conventional drugs do not work for Sundowner's Syndrome."

Observation Five: At some point, a caregiver has to weigh whether more drugs, surgeries, and other treatments are in the best interest of their patient.

Many caregivers wonder if it is even wise or compassionate to medicate elderly patients with such powerful drugs with so many potential side effects. They are faced with many questions and decisions about what might be in the best interest of their patient and his or her quality of life.

Is it any wonder, then, that caregivers struggle with this balancing act? After all, as has already been noted above, the side effects of these drugs, such as confusion, lack of sleep, and blank staring, are often the very behaviors that the drug is being administered to treat in the first place. Here are the experiences of three different caregivers around this issue.

"My grandmother is 98; she has two caregivers, one for the day and one for the nighttime. She can get mean, yet at other times, when she sees me, she completely recognizes me and is happy, awake and lucid for about five minutes. Then she goes right back into once again talking to herself. She is a big coffee drinker and they keep changing her medicine and telling her she has to stop drinking coffee. [My] question is this: How much longer do we subject her to this testing just to keep her around? Shouldn't she just be kept comfortable and happy with her foods and her coffee?"

"My dad is 83 and has been going downhill since they tried knee replacement surgery three years ago. He didn't do well in therapy and went into assisted living, and then lost the use of his legs (for some reason—they think mild stroke) and now has to be in the nursing home because he is incontinent and can't move himself. He's been sliding downhill since he went into the nursing home. Now the late afternoon/evening periods of confusion and anxiety have increased. Last night, the center called me at 10:00 P.M. because dad didn't know who his aides were—he's been on good terms with them before. I feel that dementia and Sundowners are, in my dad's case, just part of being old and drifting towards death. Is it wrong to not pursue aggressive medical treatment and just accept the dementia as part of the natural aging progression? My mom says that life in old age is so uncomfortable that people have an easier time letting go of it."

"I have refused any surgery for my mother, who is 85, and will not let her go to the hospital ever again. She is old

*enough and not afraid to die a natural death without all
the 'enhancements' the medical system throws at us. Beware!
Your elderly loved one does not have to suffer like this. Who
says they need surgery? We are only on Planet Earth for a
very short time, actually. We all leave it. Why not let it happen naturally is my thought."*

**Observation Six: Many caregivers link the onset of Sund-
owner's Syndrome with a Urinary Track Infection (UTI) or a
surgical procedure.**

Whether or not elderly patients with varying forms of dementia should be routinely subjected to major surgeries is an important question. Because of a lack of thorough research on the subject, there is, as yet, no definitive answer. However, as noted in
the previous chapter, many caregivers feel that either a UTI or a
surgical procedure in old age was the catalyst for their patient
developing the symptoms of Sundowner's Syndrome. Yet regardless of the direct causality, it is important for a caregiver to work
together with medical providers on care planning and options.
They should ask about the risks and benefits of surgeries, tests,
and hospitalization, as well as make inquiries about alternative
options and expected outcomes.

*"My Grandmother has recently been hospitalized with uri-
nary infection and suddenly today she has been diagnosed
with Sundowners. After reading all of these comments, I'm
wondering what is similar about all of these cases; [it] seems
most everyone was in the hospital when diagnosed. Could
medication or a combination of medications be the cause
of this 'sudden' reaction?"*

"On June 30, 2009, my 89-year-old father was admitted into hospital for knee surgery. The surgery went well and he was released to a rehab facility five days later. At first he was a little disoriented with all the changes in rooms and towns (the surgery was in Omaha, rehab in Manning, Iowa). But he could grasp the situation if reminded. Two days later, my dad was unable to keep a grasp of reality; he was hallucinating and seemed to recognize immediate family but talked about things that were not happening and just could not stay in the 'same' time as visitors. The doctor labeled it Sundowners; he seemed less confused in the morning, but as the day continued, he started telling stories or holding conversations that were not real."

"My 97-year-old aunt had very mild symptoms of dementia until about four or five weeks ago. She started getting very agitated, confused, hallucinating, and combative. The assisted living facility where she lived sent her to the hospital and she was diagnosed with a severe urinary tract infection. As the treatment progressed, her symptoms diminished markedly. However, the infection returned when she went back home to the facility and now she is in kidney failure. She is again combative, hallucinating, feels persecuted, confused, and the like. These symptoms are intensified in the early evening and all night. Have your loved one screened for a bladder infection. Poor toilet habits and not being hydrated can intensify dementia symptoms."

"My mother also is possibly experiencing Sundowner's Syndrome, along with other complications. About ten days ago she had erratic behavior, which included not believing she

lived in the assisted living facility she had been in for twenty months, threatening an aide, and trying to walk out. After I took her to the hospital, it was determined that she had a urinary tract infection, which was suspected to be the culprit for the sudden onset of erratic behavior. After antibiotics, she still has confusion, but no real erratic behavior. Now the confusion is considered related to Sundowners. After an upcoming trip to the doctor, maybe we will know for sure. It certainly appears that the UTI or a kidney infection can cause irregularities in behavior. Also, a friend of mine had stroke-like behavior with a UTI."

"I care for an elderly lady friend in my home. Last December, we got up one morning on the coldest day of the month to find her on the floor with literally everything all over the floor. It was a horrible sight, which looked like a crime scene if you asked me because, in falling or getting out of bed, she scraped and hit her arms and legs and they were bleeding. When I asked her what she was doing, she responded in such a way I thought for sure she was having a stroke. I called an ambulance and she was taken to the hospital and the only diagnosis they came up with was a UTI. I had been told this infection could cause confusion (major confusion) in the life of an elderly person, but I didn't believe it until I had to experience it firsthand! I don't understand it, but sure as life, that's what happens."

"Have you had your mother tested for a urinary tract infection (UTI)? Someone with a UTI can exhibit symptoms of confusion/dementia, and the symptoms do manifest quickly. I have had that experience multiple times with my

mother, when she was in rehab facilities after her stroke. (By the way, she did not have speech or memory problems from her stroke.) After receiving antibiotics, her symptoms always went away, and since she has been home with us for over a year and a half, she has not had a UTI. We also make sure my mother gets six ounces of cranberry juice a day."

What can you do?

Given all of these observations, as a caregiver of a patient with Sundowner's Syndrome, what are the things you should do to avoid some of the medication pitfalls noted in this chapter?

1) Research every drug your patient is prescribed.

Start by working with a professional who has specific experience with dementia and Sundowner's Syndrome and a knowledge of behavioral medications. Be a strong advocate in finding information on risks versus benefits. Do a Google search to find information on all the drugs your patient is taking and come prepared with questions, especially if a drug is being prescribed that is 'off label' or known to have serious side effects. Make sure that the medical providers understand your concerns. Put those concerns in writing if need be.

2) Keep a list of all of the drugs and doses prescribed for your patient.

Keep an accurate record of all your patient's current drugs (and those administered to them in the past) so that a new doctor does not re-prescribe a drug or drugs that have not worked in the past. (A spreadsheet or an online tool can be very useful here.) Include any vitamins, herbal remedies or other alternative medications the patient may be taking, as well as their alcohol consumption.

These items can have a significant effect on the way a new drug is absorbed or acts in the body.

3) Watch for potential interactions between drugs.

When a new drug is added to the mix of medications your patient is already taking, make sure that the doctor is aware of *all* those other drugs being taken. If you notice the development of negative behavior or a potential side effect after the addition of a new drug, talk to the doctor and ask to have a clinical pharmacist undertake a full review of your patient's medications. If you are not already working with a geriatric specialist, seek out a geriatric psychiatrist or neurologist specializing in dementia along with a geriatric pharmacist. (Your local Alzheimer's Association may be able to provide local contacts).

4) Be aware of dosage levels.

As we age, we metabolize medication differently. So make sure that the dosage being administered is appropriate to the patient's age, weight, and level of frailty. For instance, the research states that diazepam and chlorfiazepoxide have a half-life that is twice as long in the elderly as compared to younger individuals. This means that the drug will accumulate in unacceptable amounts in the body of an elderly patient if the dosage is not adjusted. Many other drugs have similar effects on the elderly and need to be strictly monitored. General practitioners may not fully understand elder-specific needs, especially given the complexity of dementia. Have prescriptions checked by an experienced pharmacist or a geriatric specialist, and use the Internet to create a list of questions and a baseline of education for yourself.

5) Speak up!

You are your patient's advocate. Create a stir if you feel things are not right. You know your patient and their behavior better than anyone else. Do not let someone who sees your patient for a relatively short amount of time tell you that their behavior is normal if you know it is not. Challenge inaccurate observations. The medical profession is still trying to understand Sundowner's Syndrome; your observations of and experience with the patient are important aspects of any treatment plan.

Perhaps this caregiver says it best regarding our relationship and responsibilities as caregivers.

"Please everyone, be careful of the psychotropic-mood altering medications and others that get prescribed for your elderly loved ones. Many can cause increased behaviors, falls and other side effects. Just giving a diuretic (water pill) for congestive heart failure can cause electrolyte imbalances that can send a person into symptoms of dementia. My Mom is 92 and until recently had been living alone in her home with some home health services. On Thanksgiving, she was very lethargic and had cellulitis in her leg. She has been hospitalized four times since then with a series of increased confusion episodes due to the infection process, low hemoglobin, low sodium and low potassium. Any of these can mimic dementia. She also has symptoms that are similar to Sundowner's Syndrome.... Soon after her electrolytes (potassium and sodium) were stabilized, she had no more Sundowners symptoms for many days, until her potassium got low again due to the use of the water pill with no potassium replacement prescribed. What is interesting is that she voices her episodes of 'confusion', saying she just wants it to go away.

She will say, 'I am slipping out again.' An emergency room doctor wanted to place a urinary catheter in her at one of her hospital admissions. She is normally totally continent! A catheter is the worst source of bladder infections, which can also cause dementia symptoms. Needless to say, I said no to the catheter and she remains continent and is toileted with assistance during her hospitalizations. Each elderly patient needs a strong advocate, and I feel sorry for those who have no one to look out for them; they can often get lost in the long-term care or hospital systems. [Caregiving] can be a roller coaster ride."

3

Some Approaches to Try

TO QUOTE AGAIN FROM the research article, *Sundown Syndrome in Persons With Dementia: An Update,* "Individually tailored non-pharmacological approaches for management of behavior disruptions, including sundowning, are considered to be the first-line therapy, and should be attempted before pharmacological interventions."

It would seem to many caregivers that the medical community has this backwards. Drug therapies are often the first line of intervention, with other approaches taking a distant second place. And as we have seen in the previous chapter, many of these drug therapies can have more side effects than benefits in the patients to whom they are being administered, and are often not effective therapies over the long-term. As a result, there are many posts from caregivers at the *Sundownerfacts* website that share attempts to find alternative ways to soothe their patients and create a better environment for everyone. In this chapter, we explore some of these ideas and approaches. Of course, they won't all work for you, but most of these suggestions are free or cost very little with a low level of potential negative side effects. These two factors alone make them worth trying.

Music

Music can often have a soothing effect on a patient with Sundowner's Syndrome, so it is worthwhile to experiment with playing various types of music in the afternoon and evening. Are there songs from the person's childhood or youth that they might like to hear, or that would be familiar to them? Do they like to sing along to show tunes? Did they play a musical instrument when they were younger? Perhaps that kind of music can still reach into their soul. Or what about religious music? Some Sundowner patients find comfort in the familiarity of old hymns. If your patient spoke another language in their childhood, perhaps songs in that tongue could soothe them. Try different things. Don't just turn on the radio and tune it in to the nearest music station, hoping that will calm the patient. Get creative here.

As one caregiver puts it: *"I have been in the homecare business for a long time; I have worked with clients that have Sundown's Syndrome. Try to play calm music or a jewelry box, something that's mellow and soft when they go to bed. It has helped me sometimes and is sure worth a try."*

White Noise

Some patients respond to white noise, the kind of background noise that creates a low-level distraction. Such sound is often used to help babies sleep or to aid Tinnitus sufferers. White noise also helps to filters out the sudden sounds that tend to trigger outbursts. If your patient has to nap or sleep in a noisy or busy environment, this can be quite a boon. White noise can encompass such sounds as radio static or echo sounds from nature such as birds chirping in a forest, a cascading waterfall, rain on a roof, or ocean waves crashing. Your patient might find one type of white noise significantly more soothing than another, so again, experiment. The website *www.simplynoise.com* is an excellent source for white noise. You can download various MP3 files of white noise as well as purchase apps for less than a dollar that allow you to play such noise on a range of devices.

As one caregiver noted: *"One thing that worked for me was to get a radio and turn it down very low, just enough to barely hear it. My father never liked music, but it creates noise and he doesn't wake up every couple of hours anymore. We now get five to six hours almost every night! It was a huge change almost overnight!"*

Human Touch

"A gentle voice and/or tender touch can work wonders. Gently rubbing my father's head or softly scratching his back delights him tremendously," notes one caregiver.

As Mary Ann Finch writes in her book *Care Through Touch*, "Touch is a natural and therapeutic way of being with the elderly. It is relaxing and healing, and at the same time pleasurable and sacred." Unfortunately, she adds, "Touch and its life-enhancing benefits are too frequently denied the elderly in our culture."

Touch is important. We are probably all aware of the studies which show that when newborn babies are denied the touch of other humans, they fail to thrive or even die. The elderly need our touch too. Touch is associated with positive connections to other humans, reducing the need for medications, increasing appetites, and promoting restful sleep.

Ashley Montagu, author of the groundbreaking book *Touching,* says, "The most important and neglected of these needs [of the elderly] is the need for tactile stimulation... One has only to observe the responses of older people to a caress, an embrace, a hand pat, or clasp, to appreciate how vitally necessary such experiences are for their well-being."

Recent studies indicate that massage, rubbing, stroking, or brushing the hair of a Sundowner's Syndrome patient may well have a soothing effect on them. Ironically, the Sundowners patient may receive less loving touching than other elderly patients because of their particular behaviors. Whether they are aware of it or not, many family members withdraw physical affection from a person with Sundowner's Syndrome, and this is very understandable. It is difficult to hug or caress the hand of someone who has been physically abusive to you the night before. However, withholding physical contact might make the patient more agitated over time. Some families hire a massage specialist to visit the patient at home. A late afternoon massage with essential oils can have a very calming effect. But be aware that this only appears to work when a patient is calm, or in the early stages of agitated behavior. Once they are upset or agitated, touching seems to aggravate the situation.

Redirecting Behaviors

"My eighty-nine-year-old aunt lives with me and she basically is doing well for her age. Lately she has started seeing people in her room at night, to where she comes and gets me. Last night it was about every hour. Finally I turned her TV on and that seemed to do the trick; the TV took her mind off things."

This caregiver used redirection, a very useful technique for Sundowners caregivers. And sometimes distracting a patient by redirecting their attention can work wonders. Indeed, many care-givers note that turning on the TV can distract a patient with Sundowner's Syndrome, as can playing music the patient can clap, sing, or hum along to. Other caregivers find that playing audio books, even if the patient cannot follow the plot, can work to redirect them.

Some care facilities provide the opportunity for patients to engage in repetitive behaviors that they may remember from their earlier lives. You can try this at home. Introduce activities like folding napkins or hand towels, polishing silverware, or sorting socks. If this works, keep a supply of activities on hand and 'undo' them when the patient is not watching. Purposeful activity pro-vides a focus and can relieve anxiety, especially the restless feel-ings that often accompany Sundowners. As one caregiver notes: *"My mom is ninety-six, has had dementia for several years and now has severe Sundowner's Syndrome. We have found that when she starts becoming agitated, she needs something to do to help occupy her mind and hands. Staff at the hospice facility suggested hav-ing her fold washcloths (they have a basket full of unfolded wash-cloths just for this)."*

Redirection can also refer to a more specific technique for managing agitation or preoccupation with something such as 'wanting to go home.' When the person becomes agitated about needing to do something or trying to leave, we can first validate their feelings and then try to draw them into some other activity.

This validation therapy is a technique that acknowledges the reality of the patient's feelings, regardless of the specific reality of what that person may be saying and/or believes. While this valida-tion approach may use redirection, its primary focus is on under-standing and addressing what the person is feeling. For exam-ple, we may use a *'Yes, and...'* framework to speak to the patient's concerns. For example, the patient may say, *"I want to go home!"* We respond, *"Yes, I know. Isn't home a wonderful place? Let's go over here and get our things organized while we wait."* While we may not always use the exact words 'Yes, and,' the basic concept should be the same. Validation therapy can help us better understand the underlying concerns and our support can help calm the person and reduce the occurrence of negative behaviors.

Aromatherapy

> *"I work with people that have Sundowner's Syndrome. We had a resident who had it really bad and she would be awake all night. Her family brought in a lotion that we would put on her at night and it seemed to help her sleep."*

Aromatherapy appears to calm some patients. Aroma therapists recommend lavender, citrus blends and rosemary as being particularly soothing. These all come in various forms, including diluted liquids, natural oils and lotions. Try various ways of introducing the smells to your patient. These can include spritzing their bedding and clothing, adding drops to their bathwater, washcloth, or handkerchief, massaging lotion into their skin, or using an infuser. If you use an infuser, be sure that it is electric; candles have no place in an elderly person's living space due to the possibility of starting a fire.

While the medical effects of aromatherapy are a controversial topic, it has little downside and/or negative side effects, and therefore is worth experimenting with. For further reading on the effectiveness of aromatherapy with elderly Alzheimer's patients go to the following website: *www.scienceline.org/2011/03/lavender-and-old-lace.*

Herbal Remedies

Herbs such as Ginkgo Balboa, St. John's Wort, Valerian and even vitamin E have been used to assist patients with dementia and Sundowner's Syndrome. They may or may not offer some subtle decrease in symptoms; the results seem to depend upon the particular individual. Remember that any herbal supplement has the potential to interact with prescription drugs the patient may already be taking. As a result, be sure to check with your doctor and/or pharmacist before giving your patient any herbal supplements. Some herbs like St John's Wort and Valerian can have serious interactions with prescription drugs.

Melatonin

Melatonin is a hormone that the human body produces. It plays a key role in regulating sleep and wakefulness. It has been available over the counter since the 1990s and many people, old and young, use it to treat insomnia. Some posters on the website have found that it helps with Sundowners patients, but just like the herbal remedies, melatonin has to be carefully monitored for side effects and drug interactions. Melatonin may interact negatively with high blood pressure medication, drugs that suppress the immune system, such as cyclosporine, antidepressant medication, corticosteroids (used for inflammatory conditions such as arthritis), benzodiazepines, such as diazepam (Valium) and other drugs that cause sedation, and herbs that cause sleepiness or drowsiness, such as Valerian and St. John's Wort.

Light Therapy

Sundowner's Syndrome occurs in the late afternoon, evening and on through the night. Research suggests light patterns could be part of the problem. Even within homes or hospitals, the amount of light in a room or part of a room can vary significantly. Take a good look at the amount and type of light that your patient is exposed to. Are they able to get natural sunlight every day? Is their room well-lit, with the drapes open as much as possible?

Try placing lights near a patient, in much the same way S.A.D. patients are treated. Research has found that placing a full-spectrum fluorescent lamp (between 2,500 and 5,000 lux) about three feet from, and in the field of sight of a Sundowners patient for two hours in the morning reduces agitation at night. Another study found that exposure to bright light positively affects the cognitive functioning in elderly patients. Light therapy is one approach that is endorsed by many caregivers. *"My mother has Sundowners and is up a lot, sometimes all night long. We are trying the S.A.D. bright light and it helps some."*

Reduce 'Alone Bedtime'

Many patients with Sundowner's Syndrome spend a lot of time alone in their beds. Sometimes caregivers have found that reducing the amount of time they spend there helps enormously. One caregiver found that allowing her mother to sleep with her was the key to a better night's sleep for both of them. Here's how she relates the story. *"I used to be a nurse, so I learned valuable lessons years ago that now help with my mother. I am my mother's only caregiver 24/7 and getting sleep was my hardest problem to fix. After many days with no sleep, I figured out that my mother with Alzheimer's also had Sundowner's Syndrome. I now put my mom in bed with me. When she woke me thinking it was morning, I showed her the alarm clock. She was amazed when I showed her how little time she had been asleep. It was 12:00 A.M. the first time she awoke, and 4:00 A.M. the second time. At 4:00 A.M. I gave her 10 milligrams of Melatonin. She slept the next four and a half hours without waking. I am always patient with her, but this really seemed to help. I finally got thirteen and a half hours of much needed sleep."*

Daily Routines are Essential

Routine is essential to patients with dementia and Sundowner's Syndrome. Anything that disrupts their routine is a potential minefield. While *you* may be flexible about the timing of their medical appointments, or who comes to dinner, the patient can find these changes very disruptive. As a result, like a small child, they may act out. So be very aware of creating and maintaining as much routine as possible. Group appointments together in the morning, read together after lunch, have a cup of cocoa at 7:00 P.M. These things all have the potential to keep the Sundowner's Syndrome patient calm and on track.

Here are some comments from caregivers in relation to this.

"I have had extensive experience with Alzheimer's/Dementia/Sundowner's in my job, and most especially with my grandmother. I can tell you that any change in location or routine will likely cause extreme agitation, and could cause the symptoms to worsen."

"My mom has Parkinson's disease as well, and any change at all can onset Sundowners, so keeping routine is an important key in her care."

"I have a plan. It works! About 5:00 P.M. in the afternoon, weather permissible, take him or her for a short walk. Next, turn on a lamp in his or her room, along with the TV or radio. After supper, go into their room and look at the calendar

with them and see what is coming up, such as a doctor's appointment, someone's birthday, a planned outing, go over the day ahead with them. Read the newspaper with them, look at old pictures, and right before bedtime, help them with bathroom stuff and to get into their PJ's and give them their meds. Be sure they are in the bed and leave the TV on all night; the sound will help them sleep. It has worked for us. Not every night is a good night, but this strategy is a winner for us."

Vision Issues

Some studies suggest that vision issues can play into the severity of Sundowner's Syndrome. So it's important to ask the simple question: can the person I am caring for see well? Shadows and blurry images can exacerbate a patient's feelings of agitation and disorientation. Yet when dealing with the elderly, we sometimes neglect to keep their glasses and eye prescriptions up to date (or the patient loses or mistreats his or her glasses so often that we stop encouraging their use). Particularly if the patient no longer reads, we are less inclined to think about their vision. However, getting a new pair of glasses for them or making sure they wear the ones they have may help a patient see better and reduce the potential of agitation as shadows lengthen and nighttime approaches.

Monitoring From Afar

Today we are fortunate to have a plethora of modern gadgets to help us with our daily tasks. Some of these new innovations are particularly adaptable for use with Sundowner's Syndrome patients. Perhaps the most useful of all is the so-called 'baby monitor.' This device allows the caregiver to monitor what is going on in a different part of the house. Some baby monitors have cameras attached while others just deliver audio. And if you want to take monitoring a step further, an entire house can be wired for camera surveillance. However, caregivers often struggle with guilt over invading their patient's privacy when employing such surveillance techniques: *"My mother would hate to know I was spying on her."* But, as we have already noted, Sundowner's Syndrome changes our relationship with the patient. Sometimes the use of these techniques is necessary for a patient's personal safety and for our ability to manage as caregiver. There are also a growing number of other technologies being used to help with eldercare. These technologies range from 'fall buttons' that can detect if a person has fallen, monitoring systems that sense motion (versus the sound or camera systems mentioned above) to GPS systems that can track those dementia patients who have a tendency to wander.

Simulated Presence Therapy

This therapy takes advantage of modern technology. In *Simulated Presence Therapy*, the patient is exposed to video footage of loved family members or close friends. Geriatric centers in The Netherlands have found that staging a 'one-sided' conversation and playing the footage back on an electronic devise decreased patients' agitation.

A member of the Dutch team that pioneered this approach describes how they create the videos. "We start with videotaping a spontaneous contact between the patient and a favorite family member [or close friend]. Together with the family member [or close friend], we look at which themes have a good influence on the patient. These themes are used to make a short videotape. On this tape, the family member [or close friend] talks with the patient as if it were a real conversation. We learned that it is useful to mix this with family pictures. When the tape is ready, a professional caregiver looks at it together with the patient... We have learned that they both enjoy this. It is very stimulating for the nurses to experience that the patient is calming down and coming into a better mood. The patient feels better and this positive emotion holds up for a longer period during the day."

For a caregiver with some technical knowledge about video recording (or a friend or family member with such know how), this approach is worth trying, particularly if the patient has a close relationship with a particular person and tends to 'do what they say' more often. It makes sense that showing family members, children, grandchildren, brothers and sisters, can help redirect an elderly, confused person.

Many caregivers have contributed their ideas on how they deal with their Sundowner's Syndrome patients. Not all of these suggestions will work for your patient; perhaps none will. Certainly none of them will 'cure' anyone, but they are worth exploring. Perhaps you will hit upon something that works well for your patient, or something that allows you a little more piece of mind. Continue to experiment in small ways. Try one thing at a time, so that if you detect a positive change in the patient, you will have a clearer picture of what could be contributing to it.

4

Family Dynamics

AFTER CONCERN FOR THE ongoing well-being of their patient, the next most common concern found among caregivers has to do with the family drama that unfolds around a patient with Sundowner's Syndrome. This drama plays out on a personal level as each family member reacts and responds to the Sundowners symptoms, and on a group level as family members struggle to work out the potentially volatile aspects of working together to provide the best care for the patient. These struggles take the shape of difficult questions like: Who is the primary caregiver? Who is the primary decision maker in terms of treatment? Who offers financial aid? Who supports the ones on the 'frontlines?' This is unfamiliar territory to most families, and they negotiate it to varying degrees. Some families are pushed apart by the intensity of looking after someone with Sundowner's Syndrome, while other families are drawn together with a new appreciation and love for each other. In this chapter, you will hopefully find some strategies to help you accept the diagnosis that a loved one has Sundowners, and to reach out in a positive way to those around you. However, as we will see, there is not always a guarantee that things will go well.

Are You My Mother? We all know the classic children's book, but in reality, many children of patients with Sundowner's Syndrome struggle with that question. If a person acts differently from how they did before, and often in ways that would have repulsed that same person, are they still the parent their children remember? Inappropriate and unfamiliar behavior is extremely disturbing to those who have to witness it, and who often have to intervene to try to stop it. Sometimes the struggle to equate new behaviors with a loved parent or spouse can create an overwhelming sense of sadness and despair in caregivers, as these posts note.

"My 88-year-old mother is visiting us now and we want very much for her to move in with us. She also suffers from dementia and Sundowners. I have always been close to my mom, and having her get so angry with me hurts so bad. I know that if she really knew, it would hurt her just as much. I find comfort in knowing that she will not remember what she has said the night before."

"One has to remember that this is not the same person who nurtured you for 53 years through good times and bad times. This was not my daddy. My daddy would have never punched and kicked me. (My daddy had never laid his hands on me). Listen to the professionals and remember this is not the person you knew."

"My mom just turned 87. She lived on her own and drove up to a year ago. Now she has Sundowners in her new place [assisted living]. She was the best mom, helped us with our kids, now 16, 13, 9 and 6, since the day they were born. It is very sad to see our wonderful, loving parent go through this. I am so sad to see her scared. Mom, we love you! I am sorry this has happened to you."

"I have watched my mom go from someone who was always cooking, baking and canning to now not even knowing how to scramble an egg. She walks around her house, lost and confused."

"My father-in-law just turned 88 and has been experiencing Sundowners for about a week. He has deteriorated very rapidly over a few days. He has trouble walking as he has diabetes and a balance problem. This accompanied with Sundowners is a difficult problem to handle especially at night. He was a very brilliant man and taught calculus and trigonometry in college. He also taught one of our presidents. I can tell he tries very hard to remember things, but they don't come to him very quickly. He sometimes can't remember his grandsons' or granddaughters' names that he is very close to. He has always been so kind and it is hard to see him like this."

Amid a personal sense of sadness and loss, family members struggle with working together as an effective team to help the patient. The first hurdle is getting everyone involved to understand and accept the diagnosis. Since Sundowner's Syndrome is not a widely publicized disease and not much research has been done on it, understanding the condition is a challenging proposition. Those family members who live with or near the patient are more likely to have an accurate idea of what is going on than those who live further away. And since the symptoms of Sundowner's Syndrome don't occur until later in the afternoon and on through the night, even some of those family members who live nearby may not have experienced a 'bad' episode. This can lead to misunderstanding and frustration as these other family members can tend to downplay the situation or insinuate that the nighttime caregiver is exaggerating.

"I am a 20-year-old college student and have been taking care of my 90-year-old great grandmother. It is becoming extremely hard to watch her at night because she starts seeing her son who passed away three years ago. Last night she called me in at 2:00 A.M. to 'remove' the guests who were having a 'party' in her closet. I was shocked because the closet door was closed! It took a while for the rest of the family to believe me because during the day she is perfectly fine for a 90-year-old. My family told me I was just being lazy and that I'm tired at school everyday because I talk on the phone all night! I got so fed up I told my uncle to spend the night and, sure enough, he verified these strange behaviors my great grandmother has been showing."

"My youngest brother lives more than three hours away, and he comes through once a month and spends the weekend with us, to keep my dad company. My dad, of course, is on his best behavior then! That makes me so mad!"

Those who are geographically closest to the person with

Sundowner's Syndrome are often more willing to accept that this is not the person they knew than are those who only experience the symptoms at a distance through conversation with the caregiver. Those family members who live further away may not fully understand the types and depths of challenges faced, or how different the person has become to the loved one they remember— after all, the photographs still look similar. It is vital that everyone involved understands the gravity of the situation and the stress that caring for someone with Sundowner's Syndrome puts on the caregivers. If necessary, make a video or audio recording of the patient during an episode to reinforce what you have been telling the other family members. And if the doctor has made a diagnosis, make copies of the diagnosis and send it to everyone who needs to know what is going on.

Of course, you may have to face the fact that some family members do not want to know the details, or cannot face the changes that are occurring. This is another issue altogether, but do not assume at face value that they don't want to be involved. Always give them the option of knowing. One poster on the website recounts his experience with this situation.

"I have not lived at home for over 43 years, and actually live out of state, so I only knew when I would call my father, very frequently, how he was doing. He seemed to be tired all the time and I figured it was a medication I knew he was on. [I did] not know of all the [other medications] he had in his apartment, (due to a hospitalization and subsequent diagnosis of Sundowner's Syndrome). I guess I'm feeling pretty angry right now, not [having] known, but most of the family did not want to 'upset me,' so I only recently learned how bad dad was doing."

This brings us to the stress of coordinating the care of a patient with Sundowner's Syndrome. It goes without saying that it is very taxing to deal with someone who can behave violently and erratically. Some caregiver, be they a spouse, child, or grandchild has to shoulder this burden—sometimes alone. Often, they wish they had someone to lean on.

> *"It's going to be hard to type this without any mistakes because of tears running down my face, so please forgive any errors in typing. My 80-year-old father has Sundowners. My dear mother tries her best, and I have really seen her age in the past six months. I am an only child and I wish I had siblings to lean on. At what point does one turn the care over? My mother doesn't want to do so as long as [my father] still knows her—which he does in the mornings. When do the tears stop? Do they ever?"*

> *"My dad will be 91 years old. He lives alone nearly 85-miles from me and I am the only child. Neighbors look out for him and we pay for someone to check and give him his medication for his heart problems twice each day. He gets meals on wheels as well.... Are there any other only children with difficult, often belligerent 91-year-old dads with dementia out there?"*

The truth is, family groups trying to act together to make decisions and coordinate care for a Sundowner's Syndrome patient can also run into challenges, as one poster notes.

> *"My family is huge, my mother has nine kids. And yes, it's hard to take care of one person, nine different ways!"*

This sets out the issue well—one person taken care of nine different ways. None of us make exactly the same decision as another person would make; we each have our unique perspective on the world. Serious illnesses, like Sundowner's Syndrome, create situations and conversations that do not happen under less stressful situations. Nine people will all have to struggle to understand complex medication issues and come to a consensus as to what is best for the patient. And they will have to do this again when the drugs cease to be effective, or the patient becomes uncontrollable. They may also have to learn about and accept each other's ideas about when to let a parent die, or when to refuse treatment. These are serious and sometimes volatile issues and it is no wonder that families get stressed out in dealing with them. Siblings, who have not had to agree on anything since they chose the color of their bedroom walls at ten years of age, now have to pull together under the direst circumstances. As a result, old family grudges can resurface in unflattering ways.

"My so-called baby sister had Power of Attorney and really did dad in. Her and her family moved in with dad to supposedly take care of him. She was in it for the money and what ever she could get. Her and my brother told dad that they would be there till the end and neither one are there..."

"My mom is 93 with advanced dementia. I have taken care of her for eleven years now. My brother, a doctor, does not help even though he lives close by. [Mom] is on no medication except Plavix. She has no physical problems.... She has started twitching, panting, writhing around on the bed, and being violent at night—tearing at her clothes, agitated, talking nonsense non stop. She has been seeing people for a year

or so that aren't there. I am exhausted. I can't afford to hire someone to watch her all night. I have someone watch her during the day so I can go to work. My husband is a saint, but he is at his wit's end. We can't afford six thousand a month for a nursing home, and if we could, I wouldn't do it. They would tie her in a chair, sedate her, and let her die. The doctors can't help me, as she really doesn't have any underlying medical conditions. She gets violently delusional when any dementia drugs are tried. I know no one can help me, but it feels better just talking about it!"

"My mom is 86 and has been dealing with dementia for the last several years. Now she has severe dementia—hallucinations, confusion off and on during day—and by 5:00 P.M. Sundowners almost always kicks in. Tonight was very bad—confusion, yelling, cussing, telling me to go to hell. I live with her and work at home with my job and my sisters will not help."

"My mom is 77 year old; [she has been] living with me since last September and has Sundowners. My husband and I take care of her. My grandchildren come by pretty often, but I don't want them to feel burdened (they have families and work too). My sister and her 'clan' do nothing more than call once in a blue moon. My question is this: How do I involve my sister as far as letting her know of mom's condition? And what about her helping somehow, maybe financially? We need to hire someone to come a couple of times a week to help with bathing, etc. I know [my sister] will come up with some cock-eyed excuse, like her ailments, but it's wearing all of us out. I have quit my job and my husband supports

me all the way. This situation has turned my life upside down.... My mom and dad did so much for my sister; she really does owe something!"

Few people are at their best during these situations. Caregivers for patients with Sundowner's Syndrome are usually sleep deprived and stressed out with life-changing decisions. Emotions run high. No one, including the doctor, can predict what is going to happen next. Faced with this overwhelming reality, it is only human to lash out and assign motives to another sibling's behavior. Yet despite our frustration, we must try to stay focused on the welfare of the patient.

There are some steps that can be taken to try to engage siblings in the caregiving process. Focus on what it is you really need help with. What would you want your sibling(s) to help with and why? And once you have arrived at this, state it very matter-of-factly. "I need someone to come and bath mom twice a week. I have a back issue and I cannot do it. It will cost (x) amount of money. Can you pay for that?" Or, "I need a break. I have been with dad 24/7 for eight months. Can you come and stay with him for a week in September, or pay for him to go into respite care so I can get a break?"

Stating the situation and asking for specific involvement removes all ambiguity from the situation. Now is not the time for hinting! Phrase your requests for help in such a way that your sibling will have to say 'yes' or 'no.' And if they say no, or offer an excuse, then ask them, "What can you do to help in this situation then?" Or, "we really need to find a solution to this problem, can you suggest anything else we could try?"

Of course, sometimes you may have to face the fact that your sibling(s) just don't care in the same way that you do and do not see eye-to-eye with you about what needs to be done. The person who posted the comment below found this out the hard way. He could not bear to see his grandmother go into a home, so he assumed responsibility for her. Everyone else let him do so, but then it became overwhelming for him and he found himself in a real bind. His experience illustrates the need to work hard to keep other siblings and family members feeling like they share the decision-making process and responsibility, even if you are the primary caregiver.

"I'm married with a 3-year-old boy. My wife and I are 25 and 24 years old now, after [my grandmother] moved out of state [to be near her children] we constantly got calls from the family there saying that she was becoming unstable and angry, cursing at the kids and trying to fight with everyone. They decided to try and put her in a nursing home. I got angry because I helped with my grandfather till he passed. He had the first stages of Alzheimer's. Being that I'm an EMT and my wife is a nurse, we decided that since my grandmother raised me from a baby that I should return the favor and help her out.

"So now here's the issue. It's two years since then, and having to deal with her constantly getting worse... I'm losing sleep. I had to quit my job to take care of her. She's always up all night long either drinking coffee or outside talking to herself at three in the morning. We live in apartments and had APS call on us because she told someone we're stealing her money and locking her in her room. She does help with the rent...[but] we can't afford to pay her bills and ours. Now I'm going back to work because I'm making the decision to have her put into a nursing home.

"I'm way too young to deal with this and my son doesn't need to grow up being exposed to this type of issue. Her children are more capable of handling this, but don't care about her. Sure, my wife and I have medical experience and are used to being around this type of behavior, but our jobs don't require us to live with our patients. That's a totally different ball-game. I love her dearly, but I cannot take it anymore. She raised me, yes, but now I have to raise my son."

Obviously, this young man and his wife did not anticipate the difficulty that lay ahead of them. Unfortunately, it appears as if the other family members let him take over and 'washed their hands' of the situation. This is not fair. We are all guilty of idealism at times, and might even be judgmental of those who are more pragmatic. Everyone involved in dealing with a patient with Sundowner's Syndrome needs to remember that the path they are treading is new and unpredictable. People may offer help that they do not have the resources or mental strength to deliver over the long haul. The situation is not stable. We need to have compassion for others who have made gallant attempts to help and are now floundering. Sundowners is a very difficult illness to live with, and sometimes people are overly optimistic about their ability to deal with the patient, or the patient's condition deteriorates and they need more help. Just because someone in your family stepped forward, do not assume that they can shoulder the burden alone indefinitely, even if they indicated that they could at the outset.

Sundowner's Syndrome, like dementia itself, is not a terminal illness. The *Sundown Syndrome in Persons with Dementia: An Update* report states that there is very little research data to date on the prognosis of Sundowner's Syndrome. However, according to the Alzheimer's Association, a patient with dementia typically lives for eight years after his or her symptoms become visible to others. This is a sobering statistic for a person just embarking upon the care of a patient. As you start out, one of the best things you can do for yourself is to set up regular 'check-in' points with your extended family where all aspects related to the patient's care can be discussed openly and fresh decisions made about the ongoing care. Ideally, such a check-in should occur every three months, since that is the length of time many drugs associated with Sundowner's Syndrome seem to be effective. Rather than wait for a crisis, have a telephone or Skype conference with your siblings every three months to go over where things stand. How is the patient? What does the doctor suggest doing next? How about the living arrangements; are they working for everyone concerned? How are the financial aspects going? Can anyone step up to solve a new problem, or take a turn relieving someone who needs a break? Touching base on a regular basis with family members is the best way to head off any misunderstandings.

Sometimes siblings are faced with the reality that they now have, or always have had, a different relationship with their parents than their other siblings. We must allow for this. They have different memories, along with different levels of willingness to act on their parent's behalf or use their own resources to do so. Tensions can run high when one sibling or group of siblings is expected to shoulder more of the load based upon their birth order, sex, or how well they got along with the patient in earlier times.

"All my brothers live more than an hour away from me, and rarely are able to come through and spend time with my dad. My eldest brother is in the police force and works long and irregular hours, which makes it even more difficult for him. I was the only person able to help my parents, and I

did it with all the love in my heart, especially for my mom! My dad has always been a self-centered egotist, and as he got older, he just got worse! I was also the only one, apart from my youngest brother, that could talk to him and get him to moderate his behavior."

"My mother-in-law has come to live with us, at my request, not her two sons. They want her far away from them. The history with the two boys and her (dearly) departed husband has confused me, as no one has really told me what the issues have been, other than her 'being a mean b.... their entire lives.' I have a history with her as well, although not as extensive...she has been unbelievable. I only mention this as I feel that it is affecting our (mine, as I really am her sole caretaker) abilities to be objective about the meanness that is coming through now."

"It's my younger sister and brother and me. Our older sister and her husband are not helpful at all. But you can bet when the time comes, they'll be there with their hands out to get their share of the house sale proceeds. (Sorry, that is not very nice—I know.) My daughter is good about going to visit my mother, but she tends to be a bit judgmental of my sister and I. She doesn't understand the frustration and emotions that go along with an elderly mother who is in the situation my mother is in and having to make all these decisions. We've come to words several times over this and I really hate it."

"I feel a lot of anger and it doesn't seem to be changing for me (better or worse). My brother goes to visit mom and he gets her all upset talking about finances, which my mother

then dwells on. I have to take care of the finances and I don't mind, but my brother needs to stop talking with mom about it and upsetting her. I could go on and on and on..."

Over the course of the caregiving experience, we are also faced with the fact that we have very different views on life and death than other people, even those we were raised with or by. Some people are more ready to 'let go' or have their patient hospitalized than others.

"*So here it is, 3:00 A.M. and I am all revved up from arguing with my mother. Her sleep aid has kicked in and she is finally sleeping—but I know the oxygen mask will not stay on; as soon as she can take it off, she will. She will also take off her Depends if she can, and pour her drinking water in the trash and then tell me she drank it. What I constantly pray for is the serenity to accept the things I cannot change—the loss of her mind—and the wisdom to know when I cannot change the situation. My sister-in-law says a refusal to do something, like drinking enough liquids is my mother's way of shutting down (she is 95), that she and her body are more accepting of her death than I am. And (this is the hard part) that I should just let her go. She says I should accept that this is not in my hands any longer, but I continue to fight it.*"

"*Dad is suffering from depression, which began a year ago after having double bypass surgery. I finally had to have him admitted at a psychiatric hospital. Now it seems that he has some form of dementia and Sundowners. My mother died 10 years ago and so dad is all alone. I try to do for him like she would if she could. My sister thinks that we just may have to face reality and put him in a nursing home. I am hoping the doctors will not give up on him. He is only 72 and is surely too young to be admitted to nursing care permanently."*

Safety is another issue that has the potential to create a lot of division within a family. This family is struggling with different ideas about what should be done regarding compulsive stair climbing at night.

"My father has a severe case of Sundowner's Syndrome. He is 80 years old; we live in a two-story townhouse, which has very steep stairs. I have documented him making 15 trips up and down the stairs in a row, while on sleep medication.

Recently, he fell down the last five steps. He injured his neck and wore a brace for about a month. During this time, I rearranged the living area downstairs and relocated his bed. That lasted for about a week. I made a deal with him that I would move his bed back upstairs if he would let me put a gate at the top of the stairs for his safe being and it would be latched only after all his medication had been taken and he started feeling the affect. He agreed, but now he begs me to open the gate so he can continue to travel up and down. My brothers said it was cruel to prevent him from doing this and so removed the gate. Am I supposed to let him continue to travel up and down the stairs? I am scared to death I'm going to wake up one morning and find him in a heap at the bottom of the stairs."

In a strong, committed family, everyone works together to help take care of the patient. Decisions are made in concert, and everyone 'pulls' his or her weight, contributing what they can from their resources of time, money, and expertise. However, many people do not have this kind of family and having a family member afflicted with Sundowner's Syndrome is a sure way to expose the cracks. Sometimes the issues are just too great to be resolved among so many family members and it is best for all to agree to involve professionals from outside the family and follow their suggestions/recommendations. A hospital or elder care center should be able to help you find someone used to dealing with these stressful situations.

Yes, it would be good if the issues that arise regarding care for a loved one with Sundowner's Syndrome could be easily resolved among family members. But as we have seen in this chapter, some of these issues are complex and compromise on them is a distant shore. Yet, as the caregiver, we must press on through our frustration, anger and disappointment at family members. All we can do is hope that over time, attitudes will change and some of these issues will be resolved. In the meantime, as the caregiver, we must also be mindful of our own care, and we shall look at this topic in the next chapter.

5

Caregiver Well-Being

"*WHOEVER IS READING THIS, please pray for all of us caregivers. We sometimes feel that we would rather jump off a cliff than do this another day—yet we do it another day...*"

When a patient has a condition such as Sundowner's Syndrome and other dementia issues, many professionals are focused on their care. The patient's medications are monitored and their physical and mental health is assessed at regular intervals. The focus is squarely on their well-being. But what about the person providing the day-to-day care and support for that patient? This person is often overlooked in the process. Working silently and selflessly in the background and helping things run seamlessly is seen as a virtue. But what many people do not realize until it is too late is that the caregiver can pay a high price for performing their heroic role.

In a recent report titled *A Population at Risk*, the Family Caregiver Alliance revealed that caregiving contributes to serious illness and depression. Sixteen percent of caregivers report that their health has worsened since taking on the role of caregiver, but many caregivers are not aware that their activities are taking a toll on them. For example, women who spend nine or more hours a week caring for an ill or disabled spouse increase their risk of heart disease two-fold. Elderly spousal caregivers (aged 66–96) who experience caregiving-related stress have a sixty-three percent higher mortality rate than non-caregivers of the same age. It is also estimated that about half the caregivers who care for someone with Alzheimer's disease will develop psychological distress.

Women, who comprise about two-thirds of all unpaid caregivers, seem to be the most susceptible to the negative consequences of caregiving, faring far worse than their male counterparts. Female caregivers report higher levels of depression and anxiety symptoms and lower levels of subjective well-being, life satisfaction, and physical health.

Being a caregiver is an exhausting role in which it is easy to forget that the caregiver's health and peace of mind are as important as those of the patient. Being a good caregiver, whether you are a spouse, son, daughter or whatever the relationship, does not mean that you have to run down your own health.

Most of us are familiar with the instructions given to parents before they take off in an airplane: "In the event of an emergency, an oxygen mask will appear from above. Be sure to secure your own oxygen mask first, before helping your child." The message is clear: a parent must take care of his or herself first in order to help the child. A parent who does not follow this advice and passes out midway through an emergency trying to assist their child has done neither of them a favor. So, too, for caregivers; you must make sure that you're taking care of yourself as well as your patient.

Caregiving can result in our feeling a loss of self-identity, lower levels of self-esteem, constant worry, feeling uncertain and powerless over situations. Let's look at some of the reasons that being a caregiver of a patient with Sundowner's Syndrome can be so stressful.

Why caregiving can be stressful and exhausting.

Sundowner's Syndrome patients are erratic and unpredictable.
Sundowner's Syndrome presents an ever-changing palette of behaviors. Patients can be placid during the day and uncontrollable at night. It has been described as the 'Jekyll and Hyde' disease for a reason. Looking after and being responsible for someone whose behavior is sometimes erratic and violent is exhausting.

The caregiver is required to wear many 'hats.'
A post by one veteran caregiver points out this challenge. "*Sometimes you go from being your dad's son to being his social worker, advocate; then, when you least expect it, you are the son again, and you cry again.*"
Being the caregiver to a patient with Sundowner's Syndrome casts you into a new and unfamiliar role. You have to locate resources along with learning medical terms and protocols. In short, you are thrust into a world that you probably know little about. Surveys show that almost forty percent of caregivers are involved in administering medications, injections, and other forms of medical treatment to their patients. This is incredible stressful, especially if the patient is belligerent. Even trained nurses find dealing with patients with Sundowner's Syndrome professionally challenging. How much more so do elderly, bewildered spouses, or adult children who must also care for their own families while administering care and making myriad decisions about that care and their patient each day?

Lack of information.

The *Sundown Syndrome in Persons with Dementia: An Update* report pointedly notes: "To decrease the morbidity from this specific condition [Sundowners], improve [the] patient's wellbeing, lessen caregiver burden, and delay institutionalization, further attention needs to be given to the development of a clinically operational definition of Sundown Syndrome and investigations on etiology [causes], risk factors, and effective treatment options."

Every medical paper published on Sundowner's Syndrome and, as we have already noted elsewhere in this book, there are not many of them, says that more research needs to be done. We know this; explanations and answers are very hard to come by. Every aspect of Sundowners, from its cause to its treatment, is the source of debate. And this situation makes it difficult for the caregivers who are required to make important decisions based upon insufficient information. Not only that, the caregivers of Sundowner's Syndrome patients often encounter members of the medical and social service sectors who should know about Sundowners, but do not.

Deteriorating behavior.

It is difficult to watch someone we love become increasingly delusional and behave in ways they never would have before. We are not used to 'sane' people becoming delusional, and when the delusions seem so real, it is difficult to find ways to comfort the patient.

One caregiver posted her experience of watching her mother's deteriorating behavior.

"I have been taking care of my 88-year-old mother. She was diagnosed with dementia in mid-2009. What scares me now is that, for the past two weeks, she has been talking

about two Korean boys ages three and eight. She talks in detail of their visits. At first, I just took it as a dream, but every day she tells me more about them and their family, I mean in detail. Example: their parents finally moved here from Korea, their mother has cancer, they can't wait to go to school. They go downstairs and visit my son. My mother was so worried about these boys one day that she started crying. She said they were outside and wanted me to make sure they were okay. She talks so clearly about this, not confused or disoriented. This is so real to her."

It is emotionally stressful for a caregiver to have to watch someone they have loved and cared about change before their eyes; to see them slide into delusions that can cause their behavior to become agitated, abusive, sometimes violent, and always unpredictable.

As we can see, there are many reasons why it is stressful to be a caregiver for a patient with Sundowner's Syndrome. Yet it is a reality thousands of people face day in and day out. The question is: How can a caregiver mitigate some of these stressors so that he or she does not compromise their own health and well-being? Let's look at some steps caregivers can take to help themselves.

You need sleep!

Sleep is a vital part of the equation for anyone caring for a patient with Sundowner's Syndrome. The patient is often wide-awake for long periods at night and requires extreme levels of supervision and care. In the morning, when they calm down, they fall into an exhausted sleep. But not so the caregiver...he or she often has a whole other life to attend to, children to get off to school, a home to run, a job to go to. Over time, this lack of sleep has serious consequences. Lack of sleep is not something we should try to adjust to or 'tough' out. Adequate sleep is vital to our health and our ongoing ability to fulfill our caregiving role. Sleep is at the center of our ability to function well, not an optional extra.

In the 2007 *Whitehall II Study,* British researchers looked at how sleep patterns affected the mortality rate of more than 10,000 British civil servants over two decades. The results showed that those people who cut their sleep from seven to five hours a night or less nearly doubled their risk of death *from all causes.* And if doubling the risk of death is not a strong enough cautionary tale, let's look at some of the other consequences of ignoring the human body's need for sleep. In a 1997 study by researchers at the University of Pennsylvania, people who slept less than five hours a night for seven nights felt stressed, angry, sad, and mentally exhausted.

And this lack of sleep can affect our perceptions of events. It impairs our ability to assess situations accurately and make sound judgments. Worse, lack of sleep appears to strip us of the ability to gauge just how poorly we function without sleep. Studies show that people who are sleep-deprived think they are performing well in mental alertness tests, but in reality they are functioning poorly. For this reason alone, we need to make sure that we get enough sleep: Other people are depending on us to make sound, wise decisions—decisions that should not be made in a sleep-deprived state.

Maintain ties with the outside world.

As one caregiver admonishes in a post, *"Reach out to others.... This site has been a godsend. You are not as alone as you think you are. In this day and age you do not need to be isolated..."*

Don't isolate yourself. It is easy to become overwhelmed and retreat when faced with the daunting task of caregiving for a Sundowners patient. The world can quickly narrow down to the size of the bedroom in which the patient lives. This is not necessary or healthy for anyone. Yet it takes awareness and planning to 'feel' like a human being in your own right while caring for another person.

Caring for a patient with Sundowner's Syndrome can be all-consuming, but make sure you keep some time for yourself. Anything is better than nothing in this regard. Perhaps you are rolling your eyes thinking that it would be impossible for you to take time out. But start small. Read a poem while you eat breakfast and see how many lines of it you can recite back during the day. Make a quick phone call to a friend each afternoon. Visit websites frequented by caregivers. Think of an activity that you used to enjoy and get respite care once a week so you can enjoy that activity. (See the section on respite care later in this chapter.) Research shows that yoga is a helpful way for caregivers to relieve stress. Join a prayer group, or a caregiving support group. Do whatever it takes to find ways to break out of your 'caregiving bubble' and interact with the larger world. You need a break from your patient and, most likely, they need a break from you as well.

Keep your sense of humor.

We are learning more and more about the benefits of laughter, and it turns out that laughter really is the best medicine. New studies show that laughing expands blood vessels, leading to better heart health. Laughter is also a powerful antidote to stress, pain, and conflict. Specifically, laughter has been shown to relieve muscle tension and stress for up to forty-five minutes afterwards. It decreases stress hormones and increases immune cells, which help us fight off infection and disease. Laughing also triggers the release of endorphins, the body's natural feel-good chemicals.

On a social level, laughing with another person or group of people creates connectedness and helps diffuse conflict. Humor connects us to each other, inspires hope, and keeps us focused and refreshed. At those times when we least feel like laughing, we need it the most. Try to think of some ways to boost the amount of time you spend laughing in the course of a day. What triggers your laughter? Talking to a specific person on the phone? Reading the comics in the newspaper? Seeing a funny clip on *YouTube?* Watching a comedy show on television? Whatever it is, do your best to make a little more time for that activity. Your body will reap the benefits.

Make it a priority to eat well and exercise.

Caregivers often say that they lack the time and energy to prepare proper meals or to exercise. Over half the caregivers in a national survey reported that their eating (63%) and exercising (58%) habits are worse than before they were thrust into their caregiving role. This is the wrong approach; we have to find the energy to care for ourselves. A good diet and exercise regime are not luxuries; they are what will keep your body functioning well. When your caregiving role ends, and it eventually will, what kind of shape will you be in to face your own future?

Have the courage to admit your own limitations.

While you may have agreed to become a caregiver to a patient with Sundowner's Syndrome, it is a stressful job that only becomes more difficult as time passes. Accepting the role of caregiver a month, a year, or five years ago does not mean that you cannot renegotiate your commitment. Times change, people's circumstances change, the patient's behavior will change. All of these changes provide opportunities to check in and make sure that things are still working well, and tweak those things that are not. And no matter how well-meaning family members may be, sometimes they cannot manage aging parents or spouses. We are human beings with limitations. There are simply times when professionals can do a better job of caring for an extremely difficult patient with Sundowner's Syndrome.

Two caregivers grapple with this issue in the following posts.

"How long do we suffer before we say enough and let someone better equipped take over, before we too become victims? My heart breaks for what my mother-in-law must be experiencing, and yet I find myself vacillating to the angry side of what she is doing to all of us. I can't tell what is the diseased side of her and the real her! I have been to the cardiologist numerous times now and don't want to end up leaving this world before the real reason I am going.... This sounds so mean, doesn't it? How does one deal with the 'emotional self' side of this all? I am losing me..."

"Know your limits. I should have been more realistic much earlier. I am not a super hero, I needed sleep and peace in order to function, but I put those things to one side. Now I wish I had not."

Find someone with whom you can be honest.

Caregiving requires clear thinking and emotional control. Yet at the same time, the family caregiver is watching someone they know and love deteriorate physically and mentally.

And with Sundowner's Syndrome patients in particular, the caregiver will probably be experiencing a level of verbal and/or physical abuse from their patient. This is a painful situation to be in and the caregiver needs to find some haven where he or she can let down their stoic exterior and express their true feelings. Search out a trusted friend who understands the situation you are in and will let you sit and talk and be brutally honest about your feelings.

Practice acceptance.

The Serenity Prayer could have been written for the caregivers of patients with Sundowner's Syndrome. Write the prayer out and pin to the wall!

"God grant me the serenity
to accept the things I cannot change;
courage to change the things I can;
and wisdom to know the difference."

There is so much about Sundowner's Syndrome that we cannot change but wish with all our hearts we could. Perhaps one of the most difficult challenges we will ever face in life is to accept the fact that a loved one is sinking into a mental abyss and there are only a limited number of things we can do to bring them comfort.

Get some respite care.

Respite care consists of substitute care provided to give the primary caregiver a short break. This care can be accomplished through a variety of methods, ranging from the assistance of family and friends to formal care at home, adult day care, or in an assisted care facility. For example, you may have family or friends help out during the day while you take a break or get tasks accomplished. Or a sibling may 'relieve' you for a week while you take a vacation or attend a family event. You might also hire home caregivers for such needs, or your patient could attend an adult day program or take a short stay at an assisted living facility.

Of course, as the caregiver, you may worry about how your patient will react to such a change, even if only for a short time. How will someone else handle their bizarre behaviors and calm him or her down? These are legitimate concerns that need to be addressed when preparing for respite care. Start by determining what kind of care makes the most sense and might be most successful and beneficial to you as the primary caregiver. For example, is there a family member who does well with your patient who can come to the home for a short time? Is there a local care facility with well-trained staff used to dealing with Sundowners? Take the necessary steps to prepare for the respite time. Make sure the substitute caregiver understands your patient's needs and that you have provided them with the information and tools they need.

The next consideration regarding respite care is cost. The 'formal care' options are generally fee-based. Explore different options in your area and find out about the costs. What do the fees include and what extra costs are you likely to incur? Inquire about programs to help as well. Your local aging agency may offer caregiver respite grants or support, and many Alzheimer's Association chapters also have a limited pool of funding for such needs.

Remember, although respite care is about freeing up time and space for you, the caregiver, to take a break from your challenging responsibilities, it can also be a great way to explore future care options for your patient as his or her needs change.

So there we have it. As a caregiver, your mental and physical well-being is equally, and perhaps more, important than that of your patient. You must guard your health and well-being or you will be swallowed by the stress and frustration that can come with being the caregiver of a patient with Sundowners. Some or all of the steps outlined in this chapter may be helpful to you. Follow them if they are. You may also find other things not mentioned here that help you find the right balance in your health and well-being. Whatever it is you find that works for you, make it a part of your daily or weekly routine. There will come a time when you will thank yourself for doing so.

6

Resources

RESOURCES COVER ISSUES FROM money to access to information and even reserves of neighborly good will. The chances are that if you're involved with someone who has Sundowner's Syndrome, you are going to need many different types of resources. Unfortunately, you have probably already discovered that there are few resources dedicated to patients with Sundowner's Syndrome and their caregivers. Because of this, we have included a more general array of dementia-related resources in this chapter.

Start by taking inventory of the resources you are using, along with those that you may need to search for in the future. One of the most common mistakes caregivers make is to wait until they need a particular form of help before researching and preparing for it. This is understandable; it is difficult to dwell on the idea that things might get worse, not to mention the difficulty of finding the time to do any kind of research or preparation while you are overwhelmed with what is currently going on. However, any advance planning that you can do will pay off for you in the end.

Let's assume you are caring for, or helping to care for a patient with Sundowner's Syndrome who is not in an assisted living situation. Here are some ideas to get you started thinking about available resources. Jot down anyone that comes to mind who could help you with the following:

- Who can take over if you are incapacitated due to an emergency?
- Who can offer respite care for an hour, a day, overnight, a weekend?
- Who can help decode medications and treatment plans?
- Who can work with you on financial matters?
- Who can you talk with who will allow you to 'vent'?
- Who can help you work through alternative living arrangements?

Hopefully, some of these questions are easily answered, but others may prove more difficult. Now is the time to work on filling in the gaps. If you have family members, brainstorm with them first before you start investigating on your own. It is always easier to divide and conquer. Perhaps they have resources, connections or information that you do not have access to. One family divides caring for their dad who has Sundowner's Syndrome into three areas, medications and medical appointments, day-to-day living, and night nursing. There are three sisters who live nearby, and each sister is in charge of one of these areas. This works well and they feel they're distributing the workload in a way that is best for them all.

If you don't have a supportive family, figuring out where you can find help can be challenging. The situation can raise many difficult issues, but it's worth pressing forward until you find the kinds of resources and support you need. The number one thing to do is to keep asking questions, keep asking for suggestions as to what you can do next, and who else you might be able to talk to. The 'caregiving' community is very interconnected and even if a person or organization you call cannot help, they can probably point you in the right direction. Be persistent until you get the information you need.

Family and Friends

Family and friends are the first line of defense for most people in times of trouble. Yet, as we have read in the family dynamics chapter, they can also be a major source of conflict and frustration. Sometimes this is unavoidable, but often better communication on our part can help to move things along more smoothly. Make sure you are clear on the kinds of things you need help with, and that you state your needs clearly. No one can help you if they don't know what you need help with. Don't wait for people to offer specific services. Turn those 'if you ever need anything, just ask' offers into concrete suggestions as to what a family member, friend or neighbor could do for you. If a person has indicated they would like to help, take him or her at their word. The worst that can happen is you discover they weren't sincere and start making excuses. You may be surprised at the number of people in your community who are willing to sit with a patient, help with shopping, or run errands for you. Involve as many of these people as you can from the outset. One mistake many caregivers make is to attempt to do everything themselves. This might be possible at the beginning, but fatigue sets in and challenging situations arise. Then, when the caregiver realizes they really do need help, they have set up the expectation that they can do it all themselves and no one is offering to share the burden with them. If people offer help, take it; even if you do not need it right now, chances are you will later on.

The Internet

The Internet has become the main source of information for many caregivers, often connecting them with others in the same situation. The following are some specific websites that caregivers of Sundowners patients have found useful.

Sundownerfacts.com

The numerous comments posted on this website, along with the factual information it contains, form the basis for this book. Many posters at this website have had their questions answered and found a sense of camaraderie through posting comments and reading those of others on the site. Not only do these comments provide a source of 'peer-reviewed' information, more importantly, they serve as a 'listening ear.' People feel a lot better once they get something 'off their chest.' Unfortunately, those around a caregiver can grow tired of hearing the same old 'rants' over and over. This is a bind since the caregiver's world is often so focused on the patient and his or her needs that they have little else to talk about. This is why it can be very meaningful for a caregiver to connect with other caregivers in the same situation and where everyone understands the need to 'vent' and 'ramble.'

If you have a specific question about Sundowner's Syndrome or want to join in a general conversation on the ailment, *Sundownerfacts.com* is a good place to visit. The following are some example posts from caregivers who have found a measure of help and relief just knowing someone else—a stranger no less—'got' where they were coming from.

"I am so very glad to have found this website. For ten plus years now I have had so many questions about Sund-owners, which no one could really answer for me. After reading the comments, posts and thoughts [on the website], I felt as if I'd finally found the information I had so desperately sought since 1997. My story started similarly with my great Grandma when I was in my late teens. She went for a routine heart exam, was diagnosed with

congestive heart failure and admitted to the hospital. Up until that day she was making food for herself, cleaning house, talking on the phone and paying her own bills (at age 94). After she went into the hospital, she developed Sundowner's Syndrome, which began as confusion with the time of day and progressed to forgetting our names and where she was. She began thinking she was being put on the roof at nighttime, and thought it was 1940 as she conversed with a long ago deceased friend. I asked the doctor who took care of her and some nurses about this syndrome and never could get a straight answer. They simply told me things like 'it happens with the elderly' and that it is a 'form of dementia.' I spent some time researching and reading books, but hadn't encountered anyone else [whose] relative had had Sundowner's Syndrome and Alzheimer's occur like this. This website has been a true blessing to me not only by answering my questions, but letting me know I was not alone with what I thought was a very unusual situation."

"I feel for you. I am going through the same thing with my mother after a hospital stay. She is 86 and it seems to be the age most of our parents go through this thing. I've gone through some difficult times since she developed Sundowners. I have increased her water intake and am in the process of trying full spectrum lighting. Singing with her helps, but that's one tip I know can't be helpful to everyone. She always sang in church and remembers songs. I'm hanging in there for my mom and know what you have to be going through. It's so very tough!"

"John, you're not complaining, you are venting. Big differ-
ence. That is what these forums are for—a safe place to let
it all out. So if she gets food stamps, I assume that means
she is already approved with a Medicaid card? If so, they
will pay for skilled nursing care for her. You need to get
her out of your place (especially if it's violating your lease,
among other reasons) a.s.a.p. and get her placed in a facil-
ity before her condition progresses and she gets more dif-
ficult to place. If she's already been violent with you, it's
pretty probable that she will get that way with others as
her brain deteriorates. Get her in while she's still some-
what easy for others to deal with (without sedatives and
restraints)."

"I can't thank all of you enough for your experiences with this,
the 'what you've done', the 'what works', the 'what doesn't'.
It does help, although one doesn't wish this on anyone. Not
the victim's of Sundowners, or the victims of those with
Sundowners."

Caring.com
Several posters have suggested this website in their comments. The site has some wonderful ideas on dealing with
dementia patients, although there is not much specific to Sundowner's Syndrome. Still, you will find many similar problems
and potential solutions here. The website is particularly good at
providing practical information such as how to find and apply
for government aid, and where to look for resources within
your community.

Agingwisely.com

This website contains a wide variety of general information on aging and elder care, as well as some specific articles on Alzheimer's, dementia and Sundowners.

ltcombudsman.org

The National Long-Term Care Ombudsman for your state has significant resources to help assess long-term care facilities and elderly abuse issues. You can find more information as well as a link to your state's ombudsman at this website.

alz.org

This is the website of the Alzheimer's Association. The Alzheimer's Association offers local support groups, a 24-hour, seven days a week hotline, as well as national information

Your State Area Agencies on Aging

You can find such agencies via *www.eldercare.gov* or by looking up the information in your local area. Area Agencies on Aging are private, not-for-profit entities designated by the Older Americans Act to advocate, plan, coordinate and fund a system of elder support services in their respective planning and service areas.

Medicare.gov

Information about Medicare and your patient's coverage, as well as a special section and resources for caregivers can be found at this site. If you have trouble with your patient's Medicare plan or insurance claims, most states also have a volunteer-run program that assists with senior health insurance concerns (called SHIP or SHINE typically); this group can usually be located by calling the local Area Agency on Aging.

The National Center for Biotechnology Information (www.ncbi. nlm.nih.gov)

In particular, you want to go to the 'PubMed' section of this website *(www.ncbi.nlm.nih.gov/pubmed)* which is the entrance to an immense library of medical research papers. Here you can search for specific research articles related to Sundowner's Syndrome (there aren't many), Alzheimer's and other forms of dementia. In the PubMed database, you will also find the research article, *Sundown Syndrome in Persons With Dementia: An Update*, which we have referred to and quoted from several time in this book.

Blogs

We have not been able to locate any useful blogs about Sundowner's Syndrome. Perhaps those caring for patients with Sundowners are just too exhausted to write one. Who knows, you may be inspired to start one! In a post, one caregiver highly recommends the blog *My Dad has Dementia,* which can be found at *www.caring.com/blogs/dad-has-dementia.* There are a number of other blogs related to dementia that you may find helpful and which offer techniques for managing behaviors related to your situation.

Books

The 36-Hour Day (5th edition) by Nancy Mace and Peter Rabins, published by Johns Hopkins University Press, 2011.

Of this book, one caregiver says, *"I suggest you read the 36-Hour Day. It will help you prepare if he is indeed heading towards dementia. Good luck!"*

The Tibetan Book of Living and Dying, by Sogyal Rinpoche.

Another caregiver notes, *"Face it, we are at an all time high of wanting to medically prolong life. We love and feel responsible for our elders. We don't know how to die or be prepared for death in our culture. For a real eye-opener, read 'The Tibetan Book of Living and Dying' by Sogyal Rinpoche."*

Love, Loss, and Laughter: Seeing Alzheimer's Differently, by Cathy Greenblat, published by Lyons Press, 2012.

This is a new and highly recommended book by a Professor Emerita of Sociology at Rutgers University.

Religious Organizations

If you or your family has a religious affiliation, you should be able to find some helpful resources through your church. Many religious organizations have ways to help, so contact your local church or synagogue for more information. Some churches offer parish nurses, health and information fairs, and support groups.

Specialized Medical Facilities Near You

As a caregiver, you might be lucky enough to find a medical facility that has programs you can join. Check your yellow pages and call to inquire as to what various hospitals and clinics might have to offer, or may be able to suggest. Here's what one caregiver discovered.

"We are exploring a new option we just found out about. Our University Hospital has a Cognitive Disorders Clinic that we are getting a referral from her doctor to take her to. Not only do they work with the patient, but the family as well. They offer support groups for the caregivers, and I can tell you, we need it. Mom has progressed quickly the last few months and it is taking me and my siblings by surprise at how fast things are moving."

The resource suggestions provided in this chapter should get you started on your way to building a strong and durable network of support. Caring for a patient with Sundowner's Syndrome is one of the most grueling tasks imaginable. Don't try to do it alone; involve others, do whatever you can to set up a support system for yourself and your patient—you will both need it.

7

Pay It Forward

CAREGIVERS ARE OFTEN THRUST into their role with little idea of the terrain they are traveling into. Their journey can be eye-opening, and they often recount that they had 'no idea' of the kinds of problems that can occur with Sundowner's Syndrome patients. Any time we face a new challenge in our lives, there are lessons to be learned. It seems that one lesson many caregivers carry with them is the desire to never put their own spouse or children in the same position they have been put in. They want to make sure that they plan ahead. Others are eager to help create a better future for patients with Sundowners' Syndrome and those who care for them. Despite the difficultly of their own situations, they find ways to 'pay it forward.' Paying it forward, or making sure that we do not burden our own families, along with doing something to alleviate the suffering of others in the future, can create a sense of purpose and control over future possibilities.

Make plans for *your* future.

One of the scariest things about Sundowner's Syndrome is that you, the caregiver, have plenty of time to think about what could happen to you if you were afflicted with Sundowners. This is doubly sobering since Sundowner's Syndrome likely has a genetic component and the caregiver is often a genetic relative of the patient, such as a child, grandchild, niece or nephew, making it more likely that they too will eventually be afflicted with Sundowners. Apart from looking after your own health, one thing you can do is make sure you pave the way for your own potential decline. One aspect of this is to begin talking frankly with those who might have to care for you. Explain what you have been through with your own caregiving struggles (though they will probably know all about that) and come up with practical ways to address Sundowners if it arises in your own future.

Be respectful of the next generation and do not 'hold' them to impossible promises. As one caregiver has pointed out, *"I read an article recently in AARP called 'The Promise.' In a nutshell, the article said that many of us live under a promise expressly given or implied that we would never institutionalize our loved ones 'when the time came.' This was true of myself and my parents too. But I have released my children from 'the promise.' I have made arrangements by getting long-term care insurance. I found the assisted living facility and nursing home for them where I and/or my husband want to go. I told our children in the future I/we might need to live with assistance. I told them that we do not want them to be strapped down under the burden of their parents' caretaking needs."*

Buying long-term care insurance is a wonderful idea. If your loved one has recently passed away and left you an inheritance, consider investing a part of it into your own end-of-life quality. This could be the best gift they ever gave you, and it will allow you to live knowing your future is secure.

There are also other ways to secure your future. Three documents: a living will, medical power of attorney, and power of attorney will go a long way towards making sure the 'right' thing happens to you should you be incapacitated and not able to speak or think clearly for yourself.

A Living Will

A living will and other advance directives describe your preferences regarding treatment if you are faced with a serious accident or illness. These legal documents let caregivers and other medical staff know what it is you want when you cannot speak for yourself. This is a wonderful gift to give those who have to make decisions since it helps them understand exactly what you would want to happen. As well, this cuts down on the likelihood that various family members will disagree among themselves and ensures that you get what you want.

Medical Power of Attorney

The medical power of attorney is a legal document that designates an individual, referred to as your health care agent or proxy, to make medical decisions for you in the event that you are unable to do so yourself. Do not confuse this with a general power of attorney, which authorizes someone to make financial decisions and conduct financial transactions on your behalf. Even if you have a living will, it is also best to have a medical power of attorney, as situations can arise that are not covered in the living will. One Sundowners caregiver learned that a doctor wanted to perform shock treatment on her aunt. This contingency was not covered in her aunt's living will, but because she had also named her niece as her medical power of attorney, the shock treatment was not carried out.

Power of Attorney

Making sure that someone has the ability to perform financial transactions for you is very important. Some people may wonder what this has to do with medical situations, but as a Sundowner's Syndrome caregiver, you are painfully aware of the intertwining of finances and illness. Health care is a huge business and once you contract a long-term illness like dementia and Sundowners, there are hundreds of financial decisions to be discussed and made. Ensuring that someone can access your finances and make sound decisions on your behalf is a tremendous relief to those who have to deal with the situation.

There are many stories on the website which point out the importance of these three documents. Having dealt with loved ones who have not made these provisions, people gain comfort and confidence just knowing that they will not put their own family through that same situation.

In order to make known your wishes about how you want to be cared for and who has the right to make medical and/or financial decisions for you if you are unable to do so, you will need to follow the laws in your own state. State-specific forms are available from a variety of websites, such as the *National Hospice and Palliative Care Organization*. Once you have filled out the forms, give copies to your doctor, the person you have chosen as your health care agent and your family members. Keep another copy of the forms in a safe but accessible place.

Some people find it hard to fill out forms giving another person power over them. They worry that this person might not be the best choice twenty years from now. No one knows what is going to happen in the future, so designate someone now, and revisit your decision every few years. You can always make changes in the future.

Share your expertise and experience.

Sundowner's Syndrome is a very debilitating condition to have to deal with. Once the patient has passed away, all those involved in his or her care should take a well-deserved rest. However, after a period of time, many people begin to consider the information and experience they have gained in dealing with an elderly person with Sundowner's Syndrome and want to reach out and help others. Everyone who has been through this caregiving experience has something to offer: a listening ear, a word of comfort and recognition of what others are going through, perhaps a ride to a medical appointment once a week, or once a month. Remember how these small tokens of caring meant so much to you when you needed them? If you feel the urge to use your experience to help someone else, then find a local charity that serves senior citizens. There is bound to be someone in your community who would value your assistance and contribution.

Research and Advocacy.

Approximately 45% of Americans who suffer from dementia will eventually develop Sundowner's Syndrome. That quickly adds up to being a staggeringly large number of people. Moreover, we can safely assume that for every individual with Sundowner's Syndrome, at least four other people are affected (and probably many more). In the United States, this means that a sizeable portion of the population are affected in some way by Sundowner's Syndrome. Yet as of March 2012, there appears to be *no* medical or research studies being conducted on Sundowner's Syndrome. A response from the Alzheimer's Disease Education and Referral (ADEAR) Center to an inquiry as to the state of research on Sundowner's Syndrome reads as follows:

"You requested more information on Sundowning syndrome. There have been a few clinical animal studies documenting Sundowning, but until now there has not been treatment research in laboratory animals. We were unable to locate information regarding human clinical trials investigating treatment for Sundowning."

(You can read a report on the findings of one of these few animal studies (this one involving mice) at the following web address: *http://www.sciencedaily.com/releases/2011/06/110627151716.htm*)

As one exasperated caregiver posted on the website, *"After reading what everyone here is saying, it seems hopeless. I can't imagine why they don't have a medication that would work for all of these people who are suffering. One would think that with so many people living far longer than they've lived before that research would be done to help with this debilitating illness. Especially since they're predicting so many people will get it."*

Spread the word.
Patients with Sundowner's Syndrome and their families are not well-represented by research dollars or public awareness. This is partly due to the nature of the condition. As we have learned throughout this book, there are huge challenges in diagnosing Sundowner's Syndrome as a distinct disease, and just as big hurdles in 'teasing' out the symptoms from the array of side effects and interactions of treatment drugs. There are also many 'embarrassing' aspects to Sundowners, not the least of which is the perception that the patient is 'crazy.' Yes, mental illness does still carry a stigma, and this often discourages caregivers from speaking out. The poignant posts on the *Sundownerfacts* website attest to the

reality that there is little accessible information or awareness of Sundowner's Syndrome in the public consciousness. Each one of us can do something to increase this awareness. The so-called 'celebrity' diseases like breast cancer and leukemia are always in the spotlight. Sundowner's Syndrome needs publicity to attract attention, treatment and research dollars. And this is where you come in. Everyone who has experienced having a loved one with Sundowner's Syndrome has a story to tell. Get your story out there! Don't be embarrassed or ashamed. This is an illness that needs public and private funding. If we don't agitate for that, we will be the next generation to suffer from the effects of this disease. Link to the *Sundownerfacts* website from your Facebook page; write an article for your local newspaper about your experience; talk to local civic or religious groups; donate a copy of this book in your library or lend a copy to your doctor; talk to your politicians; be available to answer questions (even if the answer is that we do not know the answer, that's why we need research dollars!)

Each one of us can do something to create a better future for ourselves and for others in regard to Sundowner's Syndrome. Let's work towards change as we do all we can to bring relief to those who suffer from this debilitating condition.

Appendix
Drug Chart

THE CHART ON THE following two pages is drawn from the material presented in *Chapter Two: Medication.* The purpose of the chart is to serve as a quick reference for you to identify the medication your patient may be taking. The drugs contained within the chart are organized by groups: *Hypnotics, Benzodiazepines, and Antipsychotics.* Under each of these groups the drugs are then listed by their generic name and by the brand names underwhich they are sold.

Drugs Used in the Treatment of Patients with Sundowner's Syndrome

Hypnotics

Generic name	Brand name
Eszopiclone	Lunesta
Zaleplon	Zonata
Zolpidem	Ambien, Ambien CR
Zopiclone	Imovane (Canada, Australia), Zimovane (UK)

Benzodiazepines

Generic name	Brand name
Alprazolam	Xanax
Clonazepam	Rivotril
Diazepam	Valium
Temazepam	Restoril
Triazolam	Halcion
Alprazolam	Paxal

Antipsychotics

Generic name	Brand name
Haloperidol	Haldol, Serenace
Droperidol	Droleptan
Chlorpromazine	Thorazine, Largactil
Fluphenazine	Prolixin
Perphenazine	Trilafon
Prochlorperazine	Compazine
Thioridazine	Mellaril, Melleril
Trifluoperazine	Stelazine
Mesoridazine	Serentil

Antipsychotics (continued)

Generic name	*Brand name*
Pericyazine	Amplan
Promazine	Sparine
Triflupromazine	Vesprin
Levomepromazine	Nozinan
Promethazine	Phenergan
Pimozide	Orap
Cyamemazine	Tercian
Chlorprothixene	Cloxan, Taractan, Truxal
Clopenthixol	Sordinol
Flupenthixol	Depixol, Fluanxol
Thiothixene	Navane
Zuclopenthixol	Cisordinol, Zyprexa, Risperdal
Quetiapine	Seroquel
Ziprasidone	Geodon
Amisulpride	Solian, Sulpitac, Amitrex, Soltus, Amazeo
Asenapine	Saphris
Paliperidone	Invega
Iloperidone	Fanapt, Fanapta, (previously known as Zomaril)
Zotepine	Nipolept, Losizopilon, Lodopin, Setous
Sertindole	Serdolect, Serlect
Lurasidone	Latuda